PUBLIC HEALTH IN ACTION

4

Community health workers: the way forward

Haile Mariam Kahssay
World Health Organization, Geneva, Switzerland
Mary E. Taylor
Dartmouth Medical School, Hanover, NH, USA
Peter A. Berman
Harvard University School of Public Health, Boston, MA, USA

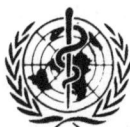

World Health Organization
Geneva
1998

WHO Library Cataloguing in Publication Data

Kahssay, Haile Mariam
   Community health workers : the way forward /
   Haile Mariam Kahssay, Mary E. Taylor,
   Peter A. Berman.
   (Public health in action ; 4)
   1. Community health aides   I. Taylor, Mary E.
   II. Berman, Peter A.   III. Series
   ISBN 92 4 156190 4   (NLM classification: W 21.5)
   ISSN 1020-1629

Designed by WHO Graphics

Typeset in Hong Kong
Printed in England
97/11665 — Best-set/Clays — 7000

Contents

CONTENTS

Introduction

The community health worker (CHW) is an integral part of many national health systems. Indeed, CHWs are essential to national health systems at all levels of development. From dispersed rural communities in Africa, to cities in Europe and North America, to the densely populated parts of Asia, CHW programmes have been established and are evolving to meet the growing health needs of large numbers of people.

Critics have claimed that CHW programmes have served their purpose and that they no longer respond to the challenge of developing sustainable health systems. As the difficulties in building strong primary health care systems have become clearer and the constraints and weaknesses in national CHW programmes recognized, health authorities and international organizations alike have sometimes been overwhelmed. Are CHWs still an essential pillar of health for all?

Measurable progress has been achieved in improving health in the world from the perspectives both of health status and of health service utilization (1). This has been accomplished through the process of development, as well as through improvement and extension of health services, including CHWs. CHWs have "shown that they can effect major changes in mortality and other indices of health status, and that in certain communities they can satisfy prominent health care needs which cannot realistically be met by other means" (2). However, as reports of governments and aid agencies indicate, even with regard to the wealthiest nations, some people and places are not reached by health services (3). In developing countries the proportion of the population without access to health services is extremely high. Whether in isolated rural villages or fast-growing urban slums, the overwhelming need for available, accessible, acceptable and affordable primary health care is the same. CHWs have been a core element in the design and delivery of health services and, perhaps more importantly, in the demand for health expressed by communities. They remain cornerstones of health policies in many countries, including Brazil, Indonesia, Nigeria, Thailand, Zimbabwe and more recently South Africa. A WHO meeting in Yangon, Myanmar, in February 1995 affirmed that most countries in Africa, Asia and Latin America have active CHW programmes. Table 1 shows the situation in the WHO's South-East Asia Region.

There is no longer any question of whether CHWs can be key agents in improving health; the question is how their potential can be realized (2). This publication looks at the contribution that CHWs make to health services around the world and attempts to show just what "the way forward" for CHWs will be.

Much of the challenge in moving forward must be met by those who implement and improve health programmes in countries, districts and communities. Nonetheless, it is important to note the continuing need for a high level of support to CHW programmes. This has been noticeably lacking from the international community in recent years. It is hoped that this volume, in addition to being useful to health authorities and health personnel, will help rekindle international support. The importance of CHW programmes to Africa has been eloquently expressed by the World Bank in its report *Better health in Africa* (4).

Community health workers: how they began

In 1978, the International Conference on Primary Health Care in Alma-Ata proposed the development of national CHW programmes as an important policy for promoting primary health care. Alma-Ata signalled a significant shift in health policy that broadened the means of improving health from the delivery of services to include social, economic and political development. Many countries had for decades workers at grass-roots level in other sectors, most significantly in agricultural extension and community development work. The concept was extended to health care and experiments with small-scale and usually nongovernmental health worker programmes were conducted successfully. The new vision after Alma-Ata was to create national CHW programmes that would serve the unmet curative, preventive and promotive needs of village communities. By their very nature, CHW programmes would encompass and promote the key principles of equity, intersectoral collaboration, community involvement, prevention, and use of appropriate technologies (5).

Today we have considerable experience of CHW programmes and evaluations have taken place that enable us to weigh and analyse their progress. Early small-scale attempts to address the problems of having only facility-based services were successful. Clinic services were reaching only a small proportion of the population, were providing curative and symptomatic care rather than preventive and promotive services that addressed the major causes of mortality, and were relatively expensive. More deliberate focus on primary health care needs was called for, with service delivery mechanisms that removed constraints for the poor and lowered overall costs (6). It was recognized that health care and drugs alone have little effect on the environmental, social and cultural factors

Table 1. Main categories of community health workers/volunteers in WHO's South-East Asia Region, by country

Country	Category	Date initiated	CHW per number of population (pop) or households (hh)	Duration of training	% of females	Numbers trained
Bangladesh	Village health volunteer	1988	1:30 hh	4 days	80	38 262
Bhutan	Village health volunteer/ worker	1978–1979	1:20–30 hh	12 days	10	1400
Democratic People's Republic of Korea	Sanitation monitor	1955	1:20–30 hh	5 days	100	N.A.
India	Village health guides	1977	1:1000 pop	3 months	25	416 724
	Anganwadi worker	1975	1:1000 pop	3 months	100	N. A.
Indonesia	Health cadre	1978	1:10 hh	3 days	100	1.8 million (1991)
Maldives	N.A.	N.A.	N.A.	N.A.	N.A.	N.A.
Myanmar	Community health worker	1977	1:1000 pop	4 weeks	5	36 358
	Auxiliary midwife	1977	1:2266 pop	6 months	100	17 856 (1994)
	Ten-household health worker	1987	1:10 hh	7 days	90	41 643 (1994)
Nepal	Female village health volunteer	1988–1989	1:400 (normal terrain) 1:250 (hill area) 1:150 (mountains)	12 days 3 days refresher yearly	100	32 000
Sri Lanka	Volunteer health worker	1975–1977	Cluster of hh	6 hours (spread out)	66	100 000 (1993)
Thailand	Village health communicator	1977–1980	1:10–15 hh	5 days		598 908
	Village health volunteer	1977–1981	1:80–150 hh	15 days		127 278 (1992)

Notes:
1. Many countries train traditional birth attendants as volunteer health workers.
2. Numbers of community health volunteers enlisted are mainly those selected and trained in the government health care system. Figures from NGOs are not included.
3. N.A. = not available.

Source: Role of health volunteers in strengthening action for health. Report of an intercountry consultation, Yangon, 20–24 February 1995. New Delhi, WHO Regional Office for South-East Asia, 1996 (unpublished document SEA/HSD/198; available on request from WHO Regional Office for South-East Asia, World Health House, Indraprastha Estate, Mahatma Gandhi Road, New Delhi 110002, India).

that cause disease and disability. Unless these factors were taken into account, it was realized, medical treatment would remain largely palliative. CHW programmes were in many cases an effective response to these fundamental issues.

The roles and responsibilities of CHWs vary considerably according to country and circumstances. In general, CHWs receive some kind of training from the formal health system to help them perform their tasks. They may also be traditional healers such as traditional birth attendants (TBAs) who have received training in safe delivery practices. In order to provide a basis for discussion, a definition confirmed by a WHO Study Group has been widely accepted: "Community health workers should be members of the communities where they work, should be selected by the communities, should be answerable to the communities for their activities, should be supported by the health system but not necessarily a part of its organization, and have shorter training than professional workers" (2).

The use of rapidly-trained health personnel, because of lack of time and resources to train adequate numbers of health service professionals, has contributed to the evolution of CHW programmes. However, it is now well recognized that CHW programmes have a role to play that can be fulfilled neither by the formal health services nor by communities alone. Ideally, the CHW combines service functions and developmental/promotional functions that are, also ideally, not just in the field of health.

The relative importance of these two functions varies according to the socioeconomic situation and the availability and accessibility of local health services. The service function is less important where there is ready access to health care facilities, whether private or public, while the developmental/promotional function is useful in all circumstances and is crucial in less developed communities.

Perhaps the most important developmental/promotional role of the CHW is to act as a bridge between the community and the formal health services in all aspects of health development. The potential of this link has often not been realized in national programmes. However, the bridging activities of CHWs may provide opportunities to increase both the effectiveness of curative and preventive services and, perhaps more importantly, community management and ownership of health-related programmes.

Linking the health sector and the community

It is important to consider CHW programmes in the context of culture, geography and socioeconomic development. Where there are few resources for the development of health system infrastructure, ways still need to be found to preserve and improve the health of the population. CHWs may be the only feasible and acceptable link between the health sector and the community that can be developed to meet the goal of improved health in the near term. In this case, national CHW programmes will be a priority within the public health system and will require a concomitant level of support. In Nepal and the United Republic of Tanzania, and in other countries of Asia and Africa, CHW programmes have developed in this way (7).

In some countries and regions, even where the health system infrastructure is developed, there remain people or places that are either underserved or difficult to serve for reasons of isolation or mistrust. CHW programmes in these situations may be smaller and more specialized than national programmes and may have lower priority. They may be targeted to specific communities and situations, and therefore require greater flexibility. In tying these programmes into the national health system, there needs to be good communication with the health centre, health care staff, supervisory personnel and the community itself. CHW programmes may be temporary, providing transitional services until infrastructure is developed, or they may be permanent solutions in some situations.

Recent developments in the USA have focused on the roles that CHWs play, or potentially could play, in that country. Box 1 gives examples of several of these developments, which include a project to investigate the viability of CHW programmes in New York City, a national study of CHW programmes, and a publication introducing the CHW approach to the health community.

BOX 1

Examples of recent CHW developments in the USA

1. The International Health Cooperation Project in New York City

The International Health Cooperation Project explores the applicability to communities in New York City of public health strategies employed in less developed countries. This project is a joint effort of the New York City Department of Health and the Medical and Health Research Association of New York City, Inc., and is supported by the Carnegie Corporation of New York. In the initial stages of the project, the New York City Department of Health worked with international health experts, local public health officials and community-based organizations to exchange information and develop strategies to address areas of public health need in New York City. The public health strategy that generated greatest interest was the use of CHWs.

In June 1997, the Department of Health sponsored a conference on *Learning from our neighbors: lessons for New York City from the developing world.* The conference, which was an information exchange on CHW programmes nationally and internationally, provided participants with the opportunity to share experiences on developing CHW programmes. Over 150 people representing a wide diversity of organizations and agencies attended the meeting. The following recommendations emerged:

- A regional version of the National Community Health Advisor Study survey (see 2 below) should be conducted to assess the scope of activities of CHWs in New York City.

- A CHW training centre should be developed to serve CHW programmes in New York City. The training centre would promote the establishment of a standard core curriculum and explore the feasibility of establishing certification for CHWs.

- Communication networks and service directories for CHWs should be developed to facilitate interaction and referrals.

- The inclusion of CHWs in staffing patterns at health care institutions and managed care organizations should be advocated.

- Technical assistance in operating CHW programmes should be provided to community-based organizations.

- A Department of Health policy workgroup on CHWs should be created to explore the role and best uses of CHWs within the Department of Health and in the community.

- A forum should be created so that public health advisors and other CHWs employed by the Department of Health can meet and share information and resources.

An advisory group has been established by the Department of Health to prioritize the conference recommendations and to develop a plan for moving the CHW agenda forward. Roles and responsibilities for implementing the recommendations will be determined by the advisory group.

Source: Information from New York City Department of Health.

2. The National Community Health Advisor Study (NCHAS)

The University of Arizona has completed a national study of the situation of CHW programmes in the USA. The recommendations of the study cover the following:

- the core role and competence of CHWs;
- career/field development for CHWs;
- CHW evaluation strategies;
- CHWs' role in the changing health care system and the special needs of youth CHWs.

The study developed an evaluation framework which proposed process and outcome measures on four levels: a) individual (CHW/client/family relationships), b) programme/organization relationships, c) community/agency relationships, and d) external linkages.

A copy of the full or summary report can be obtained from:

National Community Health Advisor Study
26 Claremont Street No. 1
Somerville, MA 02144, USA

3. Leadership brief on CHWs

In May 1997, *Community health workers: a Leadership Brief on preventive health programmes* was produced by the Civic Health Institute at Codman Square Health Center, the Harrison Institute for Public Law at Georgetown University Law Center, and the Center for Policy Alternatives. This *Leadership Brief* is a short (24 pages) but comprehensive, informative and instructive document on CHWs in the USA. It answers questions such as "what is a community health worker?" and "why CHWs?" and also includes articles on the components and results of CHW programmes, as well as profiles of such programmes. There is also information and discussion on current research and development, and on policy and funding for CHW programmes. Details of resources and CHW networks are included.

Copies of the *Leadership Brief* can be obtained from:

> The Center for Policy Alternatives
> 1875 Connecticut Avenue, NW
> Suite 710
> Washington, DC 20009
> USA

China provides a special case of a CHW programme that formed the backbone of health service delivery to millions of people in the largest national health system on earth. China's barefoot doctors made great strides in preventive health that had proven effect on mortality and morbidity. In the 1970s and 1980s, as a result of changes in economic policy and in the demand for medical care, barefoot doctors were offered the opportunity to become village doctors through training and qualifying exams. After training, these village doctors provided more sophisticated services and, in many provinces, moved to a fee-for-service financing system. Thus, a national CHW programme evolved to provide more highly trained personnel practising privately rather than under the local government. The effects of this change on utilization of curative services have varied, but preventive and promotive services have declined (8, 9).

In all situations the CHW should be an agent of change (5). Just as the CHW can provide health care, he or she can also be a catalyst for other development activities—from encouraging literacy to building awareness of basic human rights. In Nigeria, decentralization of the primary health care system to local government areas was part of a movement to increase people's participation in government (10). CHW programmes have also served both health and development purposes in Bangladesh, China and Guatemala.

Three major themes

The present study is not meant to be an exhaustive analysis of CHW programmes. It is meant to direct attention to neglected but important areas that need improvement in order for CHW programmes to make effective progress.

In 1990, the WHO interregional meeting of principal investigators, titled "Strengthening the Performance of Community Health Workers," concluded that despite the relatively rich knowledge and experience accumulated, CHW programmes were not attaining their potential as one of the "pillars for health for all" (11). The meeting recommended further study of three themes that arose from the experience of partici- pating countries but remained unaddressed in earlier reviews. These were the attitudes of health personnel and communities towards CHWs, the management and structure of district health systems, and resource allocation.

This publication examines these three themes and suggests strategies for addressing them so that national CHW programmes can contribute significantly to the sustainability of good health. In examining these issues it is important to bear in mind the context of the development of health systems in most countries. This development has largely been driven by the need to balance the financing of the pubiic health service delivery system with the commitment to equity, quality, and community participation.

Health care reform is a common theme, and the role and relative importance of NGOs, private practitioners, insurance, and drug compa- nies are changing. This influences the need for public sector CHWs and affects their roles and tasks. The concept of sustainable development and the relationship of population growth to the environment have become the centrepiece of donor and government concerns. This has led to a focus on household decision-making and behaviours and per- haps creates an even greater need for CHWs. Disease control priorities have been reassessed and are being used as the basis for reformulating national public health policy. For example, most countries in Africa must address the increasing prevalence of HIV/AIDS, tuberculosis and chloroquine-resistant malaria. The prevention and control of HIV/AIDS or malaria may require CHWs that have a single responsibility and use specialized skills.

In many places there are efforts to decentralize health system man- agement. The emphasis on strengthening district-level health systems is likely to be followed by further decentralization to county and commu- nity levels (12). This may result in more realistic and flexible CHW programmes that fit local community needs and expectations. There are also many initiatives to increase community participation by introducing cost recovery programmes in the public sector. At the operational level, concern with quality assurance and improvement, teamwork and problem-solving is changing management approaches. CHW programmes may need to become more responsive to communities as part of a result of these trends. As basic access to health services improves, the question remains as to how CHWs can contribute to more equitable outcomes in different situations.

The financial aspects of national CHW programmes, beginning with costing of the basic programme package, have often not been fully explored. Although the costs of training, remunerations and supplies are more or less known, and to varying degrees provided for, the cost of major programme elements such as health personnel time and health service resources is unknown. As the availability of resources to the health sector changes, the need for complete financial information becomes more critical and is essential to ensuring adequate support.

The three themes of attitudes towards CHWs, the management and structure of district health systems, and resource allocation must be assessed in these contexts. Strategies to improve CHW programmes and maximize their benefits must match the strategies of the health system for otherwise they risk not fulfilling their potential.

CHAPTER 1
Attitudes

CHW programmes have often started as the result of policy-makers being persuaded by a few enthusiasts. Implementation of the programmes has then been directed from the centre with little professional involvement by health personnel. In some programmes, even the health personnel who come into direct contact with CHWs daily are rarely involved in the design, planning, management and evaluation of the programmes. Although training has been provided, CHW roles and responsibilities have often exceeded what was feasible, leading to unclear expectations about their performance.

Interactions between CHWs and other health workers have been coloured by the ways in which programmes were introduced and implemented. CHWs have sometimes been seen as lowly aides who simply assist those already in clinics and health posts. Attitudes developed that did not help effective CHW performance or community links. Primary health care requires good communication, teamwork, supervision and support.

The attitudes of health personnel towards CHWs may simply reflect their attitudes to community care in general. Health professionals may not be convinced of the primary health care approach, especially when it involves preventive and promotive activities. In addition, the social, educational and cultural differences between health professionals and communities may be vast. Health professionals are often not trained or see no value in communicating with lay people about health concerns. The relationships that are developed between them may then be characterized more by distrust and cynicism, than by co-operation and respect. The end result may be decreased utilization of services by the community, and the failure of preventive and promotive activities.

If communities develop negative attitudes towards the health system they are also likely to be negative toward CHWs. Community attitudes towards health workers, including CHWs, influence care-seeking and health-related behaviour, participation in promotive activities, mobilization of local resources, and community ownership and management of CHWs.

What actions can be taken to improve the attitudes of health workers and communities towards each other? There is considerable experience from developing countries. Health authorities may:

— revise selection criteria for health professionals who will supervise and work with CHWs;

— revise curricula in medical training institutions to emphasize primary health care and the skills required for working with communities and CHWs;

— use a teamwork approach as the norm for providing health education and health care;

— use student-oriented and more interactive teaching methods in training courses;

— involve health institutions such as hospitals and health centres in efforts to increase the scope and ownership of community-oriented programmes;

— increase community participation in health by encouraging health care providers to respond to patients and communities as partners, and to improve communication;

— improve supervision of health professionals and CHWs to facilitate more effective health education and care of individuals and communities.

The vertical relationship: health personnel and CHWs

The attitude of other health service personnel towards CHWs is an important factor in enabling them to provide effective services. Most health systems are strongly hierarchical and do not provide an environment for true partnership and teamwork between different types of workers. Relationships tend to be vertical, with supervision and management that emphasize inspection and that may engender fear rather than encouragement. The problem of health personnel with "superiority complexes" has been addressed by Sanders (*13*).

This hierarchical working relationship has created several problems. There are, for instance, distinctions in status between different levels in the hierarchy, such as between the upper level of professional health workers and the lower level of para-professional health workers, and the assumption is made that some responsibilities are more valuable than others.

Hierarchical attitudes may be accentuated in the case of CHWs, who are a fairly recent category of health worker. Many CHWs also tend to think along traditional medical lines and prefer to carry out curative tasks in health facilities rather than work with families in communities (*5*). This attitude has served to devalue preventive and promotive care and has decreased the potential of the CHW as a link between the health service and the community.

CHWs were originally intended to be members of the communities

11

they serve. However, this may oversimplify the situation of CHWs who have been separated from the community by virtue of their training in modern medical care and their integration into a public health care culture. CHWs may not only take on the attitudes of their supervisors but also adopt new beliefs and expectations about health and health care. Further, if CHWs hope to be promoted within the health care system, they may become even more ardent proponents of the system's attitudes and values.

Sometimes CHWs are used as aides in health centres, clinics or hospitals, instead of as active health promoters in communities (2, 11). In some places, uncertainty about the difference between the roles of nursing staff and CHWs has even led to rivalry between these two groups. In one village in Bolivia, a feud between a local nurse and a CHW eventually affected social relations in the community as part of the population backed one and the rest backed the other.

The critical links between health personnel and CHWs are supervision and support. These have been the subject of many studies and evaluations but extensive improvement in national programmes remains to be achieved. The interest of health personnel in supervising CHWs is often minimal, particularly outside health facilities, and these personnel tend to respond first to clinical and curative demands. In many programme reviews, supervision was found to be irregular or non-existent (11, 14). In some cases, CHWs did not even know their supervisors or what they could expect from them.

Other barriers to satisfactory supervision include the social distance between health centre staff and the communities they serve. Some health centre staff may be reluctant to spend time with communities, let alone help communities take responsibility for health matters. In addition, many CHW programmes allow no time or money for supervision. This function is often expected to be tacked on, unsupported by resources, to an already full programme.

Although it is widely considered that supervision of CHWs should be a joint responsibility of the community and professional health care staff, this is rarely a feature of national programmes. The accountability of CHWs varies from place to place and generally depends on who pays them. In practice, responsibility for supervision is usually given to health care staff. Support and supervision can be greatly strengthened by designating clearly who the supervisors are and by providing the necessary time and financial resources to do the supervision properly.

Poor supervision has often been blamed for the failure of large CHW programmes. Small-scale projects are often successful because they offer supportive and regular supervision by professionals, and because they sometimes involve communities in overseeing CHWs. Such close supervision in national programmes is rare, however.

Supervision has evolved as a system of inspection with supervisors often taking on the role of inspector when reviewing CHW performance. "Performance" itself may be judged simply as record-keeping, tasks related to drug supplies and other functions which can be noted on checklists. Assessment is often cursory and may show little understanding of the need to assist and enable CHWs to carry out their responsibilities.

The attitudes of health personnel may stem partly from a lack of understanding of the purposes, objectives and value of supervision. They may also be reinforced by deficiencies in appropriate technical, clinical and administrative skills. However, health personnel should be able to communicate and educate local people, and they should, as supervisors, be able to transfer communication and education skills to CHWs.

Successful communication is highly dependent on relationships, and these in turn are defined by attitudes. If the relationship between health personnel and CHWs is hierarchical and paternalistic, communication will fail on the basis of distrust and lack of understanding, and this will be compounded by increasing lack of respect (2, 15). Without good communication essential information held by CHWs about people's beliefs, needs and expectations will be at best lost to the health system; at worst CHWs may fear supervisors and may orient their services towards perpetuating the status quo rather than improving health.

The communication and education skills of health personnel are initially developed in medical training institutions. There is a danger that the training system does not always serve to develop positive attitudes and skilled educators.

The curricula of training institutions for medical and other health sciences are not always relevant to the priority tasks that must be performed to meet the health problems of the communities (16). As a result, health professionals are not necessarily prepared to carry out a comprehensive and supportive role in providing primary health care. Despite the commitment and credence given to primary health care since the Alma-Ata conference, many young professionals are not aware of its importance and others do not value or aspire to what it recommended. One study of final year medical students in Nigeria showed that 58% of them identified community health as the pre-clinical subject they disliked most. Students also expressed doubts about the relevance of this discipline to their training as physicians (17). With such attitudes to primary health care and with little emphasis on training for the communication and education skills necessary to practise in the community, it is inevitable that attitudes towards CHWs follow suit.

The vertical relationship: health personnel and communities

The poor communications that characterize the relationship of health personnel and CHWs may also be evident in relationships between health personnel and communities (2). Chabot and Bremmers have pointed out that doctors or nurses may look down on village life, and that there is a tendency for health workers to tell village people what to do, rather than discussing with them what their options are (18).

Civil servants and administrators may also have little experience in communities and therefore be ill-prepared to communicate and respond to community needs. Officials may often believe that villagers are not capable of making wise decisions and this is the message passed down through the health system (17). Given health systems' hierarchical and centralized nature, if a change is to be effected in the attitudes of health personnel, it will have to come from the top level.

One forum for communication between communities and health workers is the village health committee (see page 28). Effective communication requires CHWs and other health workers to serve on such committees but, unfortunately, health workers have maintained a low profile, if indeed they participate at all. In one region in the United Republic of Tanzania rural medical aides and medical assistants were specifically asked to attend village health committee meetings. As villagers, these health workers could also be elected to the committees. However, this activity was not regarded as an important responsibility and health workers stayed away (19). Relationships between health personnel and villagers deteriorated and, when interviewed, chairpersons and village health committee members were very critical of local health centres and dispensaries. In some cases rural health centres were identified as empty buildings of no use.

The effects of poor health worker attitudes towards communities are significant, even in the context of curative, clinical service. Communities may become disenchanted with what they perceive as the poor quality of services, and utilization may decrease. In India, services were significantly underutilized specifically because of the condescending attitudes of health personnel (16).

The vertical relationship: attitudes of communities towards health personnel and CHWs

In the context of programme evaluations, focus groups and structured interviews have been conducted to determine community perceptions of health services and CHW performance. The information is not necessarily complete and overall appraisals of community satisfaction are not totally clear; nevertheless it is instructive to review what is known (20). Some community perceptions might also be inferred from the fact that in some situations CHWs have been harassed or killed.

Communities that have no other access to care value the delivery of services by CHWs. Satisfaction has been reported in Colombia, Indonesia and the United Republic of Tanzania (21). Even if services are clinic-based, the efforts of the CHWs are appreciated, as among communities with family welfare educators in Botswana (22). However, while some communities report positive attitudes, there are few concrete examples of ongoing support and encouragement. Instead, many communities report dissatisfaction and frustration with the limited range of services CHWs can provide, and they are especially critical of deficiencies such as lack of medicines and limited referral.

The variation between CHW programme intentions and community perceptions may be due partly to political and social influences, and partly to the fact that diverse communities generate differing expectations. While it may not be possible to generalize from specific situations, the importance of community perceptions should not be underestimated where a programme is aiming for increased participation and sustainability.

Changing attitudes

It should be clear that if primary health care and CHW programmes are to succeed a process of attitudinal change among health workers at all levels is urgently needed. There are several ways to begin this process.

Revising selection criteria

The WHO Study Group recommended that governments establish their own selection guidelines for CHWs in the light of the kind of CHW programme that best suits each country's needs and resources. If the CHW programme relies mainly on briefly trained, part-time volunteers, selection might emphasize qualities such as acceptability to the community and motivation more than educational attainment. However, if CHWs are to perform a wide range of services and to receive correspondingly longer training, selection guidelines will need to refer also to learning ability.

Since CHWs are expected to influence the attitudes and practices of communities sufficiently and in such ways as to improve health, key attributes might be social standing, a long-term commitment to the community to be served, and an ability to influence by word and example key sections of the community, particularly mothers.

As a working principle, formal selection criteria should not override community choice and local circumstances. Since it is important for a CHW to be acceptable to the community, the community must be fully involved in selecting the CHW, though health service personnel must adequately prepare the community to make the selection. The functions and roles of CHWs, and the expectations the community has of them, must be fully discussed and agreed upon. This will ensure that the community understands the selection criteria and, together with the health professionals, can use these criteria to choose the most suitable candidate.

Although much has been written about the appropriate selection of CHWs, there has been little consideration of how health workers above this level are selected for formal training in the national health system. Most countries rely on educational attainment and formal examinations. Although there are some attempts to achieve geographic, ethnic and gender representation, there are few, if any, examples of consideration of factors that might more accurately reflect attitudes towards health care approaches or towards communities. It is reasonable to assume that many attitudes are established through training and practice, but health personnel come to their chosen career with many attitudes already formed. Are there criteria for selection that would help choose trainees who are predisposed to the practice of primary health care? If so, it might be appropriate to amend selection procedures to include them.

Revising curricula

Training curricula for both basic and continuing education of health care workers should provide adequate orientation to primary health care and skills that are relevant for work in the community. The skills needed for assessing community problems and developing and managing primary health care programmes are often not emphasized, or are not present, in training programmes.

In addition to the medical or technical aspects of health, training must provide an understanding of primary health care. This will include knowledge of environmental, psychological, economic, cultural and social factors that affect health. This implies that there must be study of the social and behavioural sciences as well as the life sciences. The resulting health care approach should not just be oriented to curing diseases but should see medicine also as a social science (23).

During their training, students need to be actively involved in health care in the community, working with teachers who can demonstrate interpersonal communication with community members. This will sensitize students at an early stage to the different health and social problems of the population and will help them develop a more practical appreciation of community life. Boxes 2, 3 and 4 describe how this kind of training is given to medical students in Mexico, Zimbabwe and India.

Using a teamwork approach

Different categories of health personnel must learn to work together. Since the different categories are trained separately they are not always

BOX 2

Community-oriented medical training

Mexico

The autonomous metropolitan university in Mexico City has adopted community-oriented health care training for physicians. The medical curriculum consists of a series of 12-week modules. Each module is oriented to a particular problem or issue and includes material from disciplines such as epidemiology, sociology, psychology, anthropology and economics. The training programme emphasizes community experience.

In many cases, the medical students work with students of nursing, pharmacology, social work, community or urban planning, and agronomy. Their tasks often involve analysing the health problems of specific communities, using data gathered in neighbourhoods, workplaces and schools, in order to propose solutions.

The students spend their fifth year of study in a rural setting where they are visited regularly by faculty members. During this period, they help to develop programmes for adult or school health. Students are assessed not only on the adequacy of their clinical management but also on their success in helping to establish a community health committee and, sometimes, on changes in health indicators.

Source: Braveman and Mora (*24*).

BOX 3

Changing attitudes in medical students

Zimbabwe

Attitude change is addressed by the University of Zimbabwe Medical School in Harare where many students have been negatively inclined towards community medicine. A debate about curriculum reform is under way. Meanwhile, a project which aims at orienting fourth-year students in child health towards primary health care is undertaken annually. During the 12-week part of the project which deals with paediatrics, all students spend two weeks in a rural district hospital rather than in a hospital in Harare. Up until this point, most students have had little or no contact with rural areas during their training. The main goals of the paediatric section of the project are: to illustrate high childhood disease prevalence in rural areas and reveal its causes; to introduce students to the services available to combat these diseases; to demonstrate primary health care, and particularly the interaction of health with other aspects of development; and to give students practical experience in a low technology environment.

As well as spending time at the district hospital, students also participate in work at rural health clinics and in villages. They meet village health workers and development workers from other sectors and also attend health committee meetings. During this period, students also undertake a project related to primary health care.

Source: Waterston and Sanders (*25*).

BOX 4

Training primary healh care doctors

India

The Chiristian Medical College and Hospital at Vellore has developed a programme that aims to train "basic doctors" who can function in any setting. The training has four phases.

Phase 1. On entering medical school, the students are introduced to sociology, psychology and biostatistics. To become familiar with the demographic, social, economic and environmental aspects of rural community health as well as the role of various members of the health team, the students, in groups of two or three, live for two weeks in a community. Each group is assigned 12–15 households to study in detail. To interact effectively with the community, the students also organize and participate in activities such as health education, immunization programmes, construction of pit latrines, and management of simple clinics. In these activities they work with community leaders and other health workers.

Phase 2. This phase takes place during the first clinical year and lasts for two weeks. It focuses on the principles of epidemiology, health administration and health planning. The students, in groups of 10–12, undertake field investigations on morbidity and mortality in two or three villages. On the basis of lectures and the data they have gathered, the students plan a programme for a defined problem in a specific population.

Phase 3. The third phase takes place during the second clinical year and lasts for two to three weeks. The purpose is to give the students an opportunity to practice the knowledge and skills they have acquired in the two previous phases. Groups of five or six students evaluate the health status of a community of 1500 inhabitants and then plan, implement and assess a programme. Staff members from the college are available if the students need guidance. Phase 3 ends with an evaluation of the students' change in attitude to rural medical care and of the knowledge acquired as a result of the programme, as well as an assessment of the programme by the students themselves.

Phase 4. The one-year compulsory internship includes a three-month community health posting which aims to prepare the interns as "basic doctors". During this period they are members of the health team and participate in the organization and implementation of a primary health care programme. They also conduct studies to assess the health status of the community.

Source: Joseph (*26*).

prepared to work effectively in health care teams. To do so, health workers need training in working with other care providers (*16*). The teamwork approach will lay the foundation for increased solidarity and respect among health care workers. They will realize that they are interdependent but that they share responsibilities and need to interact frequently.

At district and community levels, intersectoral coordination is an important pillar of primary health care. Given the multiple causes of health and disease, the team concept must be expanded even beyond the health care workers. To enhance the understanding of development and to strengthen preventive and promotive activities, community teams should include workers from sectors such as agriculture, water supply, education and housing.

Using student-oriented teaching methods

To carry out their responsibilities, especially at the periphery, health workers must learn from and negotiate with communities. They must assess the local situation in its broadest context and devise strategies for applying resources so that they have the greatest effect on health. Health workers need to provide leadership and vision, and to take part in effective decision-making about activities and programmes. However, traditional teaching and learning methods are still used in many health training institutions. Students who are passive recipients of large amounts of information that must be memorized will be ill-prepared for critical thinking and independent work.

Training institutions need to make greater use of problem-solving teaching approaches in which students are asked to collect and analyse information in actual situations and to devise and implement reasonable solutions (23). Teachers become tutors, mentors and resource persons who are equally involved in problem resolution. This more horizontal approach requires different patterns of communication and interaction between students and teachers. If students are encouraged and expected to be active participants and to interact substantively with their teachers, later on they will be more likely to see both their supervisors and their subordinates as colleagues and collaborators.

Involving health institutions

Although training institutions are the logical starting point for changing health worker attitudes, the institutions that deliver primary health care on a regular basis provide the best opportunities for reinforcing changes. Health worker attitudes can be influenced through in-service or on-the-job training, by the example of more senior or more highly trained care providers, and by the vision and values expressed by the institution's leaders. If an organization's vision reflects positive and enabling attitudes, and if it is communicated to and understood by all staff, it may help determine how health personnel will think and act with regard to CHWs and communities.

On-the-job training is increasingly emphasized in many primary health care programmes both because of the need to update and upgrade health care workers in a rapidly changing field and because of the desire to improve the quality of services. In-service training may be more efficient than formal training courses. It provides an opportunity to apply knowledge and skills in a practical setting and to adapt them to the local situation. Along with knowledge and skills, attitudes are taught, modelled and encouraged during on-the-job training, although they may not be specifically emphasized.

In the context of decentralization, it is probably most useful to involve health care institutions in changing the attitudes of health personnel and CHWs at district level and below. The district hospital is expected to play an essential role in primary health care, although there is evidence that few district hospitals have assumed this role (27). However, along with its associated health posts and clinics, the district hospital forms the basic infrastructure of most primary health care systems.

If hospitals and health posts are to contribute to changing health worker attitudes, there probably needs to be a culture change within many institutions. This may be achieved through quality improvement programmes with strong institutional leadership. As these programmes develop, and as they extend through teamwork to improving the delivery of care, specific activities of hospitals and health posts can be changed. This will lay the foundation for improving both day-to-day role modelling of positive attitudes as well as more formal on-the-job training. It is likely that these changes will be made in the context of strengthening district health systems.

Increasing community participation

While health worker attitudes towards communities may be improved through better understanding of and commitment to primary health care, sustainable benefits may not be achieved until there is ongoing communication of needs and expectations between communities and health services. Ways of establishing understanding and communication vary according to the situation. Several mechanisms for communication have been discussed in the past, such as village health committees or development committees. These have not always been empowered or expected to function as true partners with the health system, but they may contribute to the development of attitudes on both sides. Potential changes relating to this kind of group are discussed below (page 28).

Identifying precisely what the community expects from primary health care and what it thinks about the quality of current services might help national CHW programmes to better understand community attitudes. Primary health care services exist to improve the health of individuals and communities; participation of these individuals and communities in their own health care (whether by patients returning for refills of tuberculosis medicines or by community use of latrines) is essential to improving health outcomes. As customers of CHWs and other health services, what do communities want? How are these wants used to design and implement effective health services?

The importance of understanding the individual or community as a customer of health services cannot be overstated. The biggest current challenge to CHW programmes is to establish an awareness of this among health workers. Once this awareness is established through training and experience, changes may eventually be needed in the health system to enable these health workers to adapt services accordingly.

The second challenge is for CHW programmes to use information on community expectations and judgements in a valid and cost-effective manner. The contribution of family planning programmes to the understanding of "client satisfaction" may be useful in this context. National CHW programmes can collect and utilize information about services on an ongoing basis through health facilities and the health development structure (see page 46). While tools such as simple questionnaires and focus group guidelines exist, training of programme managers and supervisors may be necessary to make the best use of information collected.

Improving supervision

There must be clear strategies for supervision. These need to be learned (e.g. in workshops on supervision at district level) so that professionals and community members know what is expected of them as supervisors. Guidelines for supervision should include a list of supervisory activities and details of stocks to be checked, as well as ways of ensuring that difficulties in case management and referral are brought to light and discussed.

With regard to changing the attitudes of health personnel, CHWs and communities, perhaps the greatest improvement will result from improving communication in the supervisory process. Efforts to improve communication through training and the role model of supervisors have been successful in small-scale programmes. The challenge that remains is to expand these successes to national programmes.

Training institutions and health services set the example

Progressive training institutions, local hospitals and health centres have already taken action to enhance primary health care and bring about attitude change. New training approaches and curricula have been tested in long-term courses, seminars, workshops and outreach programmes. It is not possible to describe all the improvements and achievements in health worker training. However, the following examples illustrate opportunities for change.

At the Jimma School of Health Sciences in Ethiopia, physicians, nurses and other health workers are trained as teams in a community-oriented training programme. During the training period, teams live in villages in order to assess various health and social problems through action-oriented research. This training approach is expected to improve community health and CHW programmes (11).

Efforts have also been made to develop more positive attitudes among CHWs in established programmes. In 1988 in the Maldives, workshop activities were conducted with family health workers to identify the knowledge, skills and attitudes required to carry out specified tasks relating to community concerns, primary health care and problems encountered in the field. The attitudes of participants towards communities and other health workers improved greatly as the result of focused discussion and working out solutions to their own problems (11).

Several countries in Latin America have developed programmes to train physicians for community-oriented primary health care. Traditional medical curricula were revised to include the application of epidemiological tools to analyse community health problems, local health care administration and planning, community participation, exposure to nonmedical disciplines needed for primary health care, and the use of innovative learning methods such as problem-solving in multidisciplinary teams (11).

There are numerous church-administered and nongovernmental hospitals at district and local levels that have initiated CHW activities or more comprehensive community outreach programmes. Many of these small-scale programmes are very successful. Project staff appear to have more effective partnerships with communities and CHWs than do staff of national public health services. Examples of such outreach programmes are those of the Tenwek Hospital in Kenya, the Mvumi Hospital in the United Republic of Tanzania, the King Edward Memorial Hospital in India, and the Dr Carlos Luis Valverde Vega Hospital in Costa Rica (27, 28, 29, 30). The Costa Rican programme is described in Box 5.

An important role of hospitals is to mobilize the community for participation in primary health care through dialogue with leaders and community members as well as through the promotion of community health committees. Hospitals also conduct health worker training, establish health posts, provide curative and preventive care, offer health education, initiate intersectoral collaboration, involve various interest groups in health, and carry out focused programmes such as maternal and child health or family planning. Although health professionals who have previously been involved only in hospital care may not find such outreach programmes easy to implement, the programmes greatly extend the effectiveness of health care services.

BOX 5

"The hospital without walls"

Costa Rica

In the 1950s, the Dr Carlos Luis Valverde Vega Hospital in San Ramon, Alajuela, Costa Rica, introduced the "hospital without walls" programme. Despite opposition from the medical establishment and others the programme has had some remarkable achievements.

The hospital has a clear philosophy: successful health action is measured not just by what is done inside the hospital but, more importantly, by the initiatives taken within the hospital's area of influence. Consequently, it is the hospital's responsibility to extend health activities beyond its own walls. This calls for dedication not only to curative and preventive medicine but also to an understanding that the latter is above all a matter for individuals and communities. The hospital aims to improve the health and living standards of the population by also becoming involved in activities relating to such matters as housing, land tenure, electricity supply, drinking-water and roads.

Working through, and with, five health centres, five social security clinics and 46 health posts (which it helped to establish) throughout the area, the hospital has helped raise living standards, has developed active community participation in the provision of health care, and has provided appropriate training for professional staff and community workers.

Source: Paine and Siem Tjam (27).

Signs of change

The attitude change in favour of primary health care is not easy to introduce. It is a slow process and, for many health professionals, it may be a painful experience as they delegate many traditional tasks to health workers with shorter training.

However, enlightened politicians, managers and health professionals have understood that more democratic approaches to health care are necessary if a true improvement in the health status of the population at large is to be achieved. These people have at times taken courageous initiatives to introduce change, be it with regard to health policy, health service structure, training programmes or the direct delivery of health care. Box 6 describes how the health system in Zimbabwe was restructured along the lines of primary health care.

Although change is slow, there are signs that younger generations of health professionals—particularly those who have followed community-oriented training programmes—are gaining a better understanding of public health problems and are showing greater concern for community health. Increasingly communities are determining what they want from health care, if not how to achieve it. The development of more cooperative and collaborative attitudes from all sides, beginning with the successful approaches already identified, may speed the evolution of primary health care.

BOX 6

Restructuring the health system in line with primary health care

Zimbabwe

In line with the primary health care approach, the delivery and management of health care at all levels have been transformed. Curative and preventive services have been integrated and provincial and district health teams established with representatives of all the major agencies providing health care as well as from other sectors and the relevant local government structures. The hospital doctor no longer has only a curative role but is responsible for mobilizing, through the health team, health promotive, preventive, curative and rehabilitative services, and for training new groups of health workers and ensuring integration with other sectors. Reforms have been made in medical and nursing education and in the training of other health workers.

Source: Sanders (*13*).

CHAPTER 2
Structure and management

The level of the health care system most suited to support primary health care programmes is commonly agreed to be the district. District health systems facilitate coordination and collaboration between local and national levels of health services. Although district health systems vary from country to country, the WHO Global Programme Committee has provided a broad definition which applies to most health systems.

> A district health system based on primary health care is a more or less self-contained segment of the national health system. It comprises first and foremost a well-defined population, living within a clearly delineated administrative and geographical area, whether urban or rural. It includes all institutions and individuals providing health care in the district, whether governmental, social security, nongovernmental, private, or traditional. A district health system, therefore, consists of a large variety of interrelated elements that contribute to health in homes, schools, work places, and communities, through the health and other related sectors. It includes self-care and all health care workers and facilities, up to and including the hospital at the first referral level and the appropriate laboratory, other diagnostic, and logistic support services. Its component elements need to be well coordinated by an officer assigned to this function in order to draw together all these elements and institutions into a fully comprehensive range of promotive, preventive, curative and rehabilitative health activities (12).

There is widespread agreement that the strengthening of district health systems based on primary health care is key to improving CHW programmes. The 1986 Yaoundé Conference held this to be self-evident (31).

The district health system is the support framework that the CHW must have in order to function effectively and without which the CHW scheme may fail. This support should combine supportive supervision and systematic training of practising CHWs with a reliable referral system, technical assistance, a supply system and an information system.

If the district health system is weak, CHW programmes often experience problems in areas such as supply and supervision. In order to improve CHW programmes, the WHO interregional meeting on Strengthening the Performance of Community Health Workers identified three components of the district health system that need attention: the health service structure, the health management structure, and the health development structure. These components include facilities, personnel and representative groups as follows (*32*):

Health service structure:
— district hospitals
— health centres
— health posts.

Health management structure:
— district medical/health officers
— heads of district hospitals
— heads of health centres
— heads of health posts.

Health development structure:
— district councils, health committees, development committees
— subdistrict councils, committees
— community/village councils, health committees
— special-purpose or interest groups, both formal (farmers' groups, labour groups) or informal (women's groups, family groups), which may not recognize their contribution to health development.

Most evaluations and studies of the district health system have focused on the health service structure and the health management structure. These two components include the elements that support the main functions of CHW programme implementation such as selection, training, supervision, logistics and supply, and remuneration. Although many countries have taken action to strengthen these functions, problems persist and many CHW programmes have failed to be maintained or sustained. In striving for sustainability, the focus has been on the traditional structures of health services and health management. Administrators have not utilized the health development structure to any great extent and may not fully understand its potential. Building effective partnerships with communities through this structure may be an important key to improving and sustaining CHW programmes in the future.

"Partnerships" are functional links between the different parties involved in health-related matters outside the formal health system and those within the district primary health care system. Those outside the formal health system might include village councils and committees, interest groups, civic organizations and other groups whose activities have a bearing on health. These groups may be specifically health-related or they may have a mandate in areas such as education, agriculture, water supply or economic development. The furtherance of good health and the prevention of ill-health will not occur without partnerships between all parties. This has been the hallmark of small, non-governmental primary health care programmes that have supported CHWs successfully.

The functions of the health development structure, especially village health committees, range from coordination to decision-making. Strengthening of this structure is necessary not only for CHW programmes but also for improving district health systems in general. The characteristics thought to be necessary for the success of district health systems—such as decentralization, integration, efficiency, equity and quality—all depend on interaction with communities.

Little attention has been paid at national and district levels to the health development structure. There have been reports on the role and organization of village health committees but they have seldom been analysed as components of a structural framework. In response to the need for more detailed information, WHO supported a cooperative study to describe and analyse health development structures within the district health system in Colombia, Indonesia, Jamaica, Nigeria, Philippines, Senegal, Sudan and Yemen, and to assess their contribution to health development within these systems (32). The survey in Nigeria is described in Box 7.

The study first revealed the need to describe the health development structure more explicitly and to include organizations that make up the structure as well as their functions. A health development structure is a network of organizations, and the people within them,[1] with an interest in promoting the health and well-being of a given community. It is not concerned with health policies about illness and disease. The key findings of this study were:

- There are many different models of health development structures.
- The activities of the health development structure which contribute to health are varied and include health service activity, management of health services, local planning and policy development, the provision of social and physical infrastructure to promote health and the encouragement of collaboration across sectors.

---

[1] Since the term "civil society" has recently been widely used to describe the health development structure, the expression "civil society organizations for health" could also be used here.

BOX 7

Health development structures: how are they working?

Nigeria

The survey in Odogbolu, Ogun State, found that health development structures (community development councils, primary health care management
committees, the Better Life Programme, social clubs, cooperative societies,
religious groups, traditional organizations) could serve as useful links for the
effective functioning of primary health care. The health development structures
with the most effect at village level are the village health committees. These
committees are now found in almost all the 100 communities in the local
government area where they have been very active in promoting primary
health care activities. Latrines, mosquito nets, deep wells and sanitation have
been provided and voluntary health workers identified thanks to the village
health committees.

The community development council maintains slaughter houses and con-
structs community drainage and multipurpose community facilities. Although
the Better Life Programme is involved in cottage industries, its activities can
also have an impact on health. The Programme has built maternity centres,
provided drugs and food and promoted the hygienic preparation of food.

More than half of the religious, youth and social clubs included in the survey
had no activities relating to health. It appears that many of these groups had
not been properly educated about the need for community participation for
health. The school survey showed that there were no clubs or committees
responsible for the promotion of health in schools.

Source: The role of civil society in district health systems: hidden resources (*32*).

- The operation and effectiveness of the health development structure are influenced by resource availability, health sector coordination, the representativeness of the structure, the skills for
  collaboration within the community and among health sector
  personnel, and the level of political and administrative support
  for the structures.
- Health development structures outside the formal health sector
  are an invisible resource for health development that could be
  utilized to great effect.

Village health committees: the formal link

At the local level, the health development structure includes all community members. However, health care providers (and other development
workers) are not usually in direct contact with everyone in a village.
Communication takes place either on an individual level between health
worker and patient or on the community level with recognized groups
that represent the population in some way. These groups can include
village councils, health and other development committees, groups of

village elders, farmers' and labour organizations, societies of traditional healers, or special interest groups such as women's associations or religious groups.

Most communities have councils—whether traditional or modern, elected or appointed—that attend to the administration of community matters. In some communities the council may be responsible for health development, while in others there may be a general development committee that oversees activities in various sectors, including health. However, it is commonest for health to be assigned to a special health committee. The village health committee, which is responsible for making decisions regarding health on behalf of the community, is thought to be the most important group in the health development structure.

Village health committees reflect the needs of the people and help the community to look after its health. There may be variation in the tasks of village health committees in different communities, but in general they collect information, identify needs and problems, identify solutions and plans for achieving them, establish priorities, obtain resources, carry out plans in collaboration with health workers, mobilize the community, and communicate results (33). Village health committees are a source of support for CHWs and CHW activities such as immunization, environmental sanitation campaigns, collection of information and reporting, management of essential drug schemes, organization of transport for referrals, and remuneration of volunteers (34).

Village health committees may be appointed by the village council or elected by the community. The size of the committee varies from place to place and representation may be intentionally wide or narrow. In general committees have 5–8 members and include political and religious leaders, representatives of interest groups and in some places local health workers. Though the structure may vary, the committee must be capable and must have the confidence of the population in order to be effective.

The village health committee must interact both with various groups and people in the community and with the health care system. The extent to which the committee interacts with and represents the community will determine the extent of local participation. It is important to define what we mean by "community". In some countries communities are clearly defined by geography and ethnic group, and are highly organized. In other places, villagers may be linked only by physical proximity and may not act as a cohesive unit. Communities may be defined more by occupation, religion, class or caste, or ethnic group. With increasing migration to urban areas, mixed communities may be the norm. These differences influence the roles and potential effectiveness of committee representatives.

Since district health systems, including CHW programmes, are nearly always organized geographically, the tendency is to establish health committees by geographic area too. This may be essential for effective interaction with the health system but may have a negative impact on community development. Like CHWs, village health committees are intended to bridge the gap between primary health care services and communities. It is important to remember that this bridge spans not only different beliefs and experiences but also different social organizations.

In one Zambian programme, 83% of CHWs reported that village health committees had been formed, of which about half met monthly and another quarter met every three months (11). In some studies, CHW performance has been shown to be positively associated with the level of support from village health committee activities. For example, a study in Nigeria identified support and encouragement by the village health committee as an important factor in CHW job satisfaction (14). In Ecuador, the presence of a health committee was strongly associated with superior CHW performance in the areas of prevention and maternal-child health (35).

In many other programmes, however, health committees are weak, inactive or moribund, formed because they were part of a workplan but never encouraged. Community support may be lacking and links with the health sector may be limited (29). Reviews have shown that the process of developing village health committees has often been poorly planned and executed. It would therefore be premature to dismiss them as ineffective if they have not been correctly implemented.

Reviewing the problems and constraints of village health committees can help in assessing potential capabilities. Many committees have not been able to support, supervise or collaborate with CHWs, nor have they been able to collect funds to pay them (36). In a Tanzanian programme village health committees restricted themselves to countersigning CHWs' monthly reports. A more detailed study of Kenyan village health committees showed that there was no communication between committees and project management. This led to conflicts when decisions that affected villages came to be implemented.

Representation

Village health committees may not be representative of the entire population. Important minorities and vulnerable subpopulations may be excluded, as is often the case with women, and especially young mothers. The very poor may not be represented, even though they may have the greatest need for services. The fact that communities are usually not homogeneous entities even though they share a common geographic territory is often not allowed for during the process of selecting committee members. Even when some attempt is made to include subgroups such as women, traditional power structures may influence participation. Cultural and socioeconomic factors often divide communities into distinct and conflicting interest groups (17). There is a risk that the more powerful, influential and wealthy groups will monopolize community councils and health committees (37). Many community participation projects have failed because they did not take class interests in communities into consideration. They worked only through community leaders who often had their own interests at heart (38).

Lack of representativeness of health committees has also tended to result in inappropriate selection of CHWs. Jobs become resources to be allocated (whether for salary, status, or other benefits). In some countries it was found that the sons, daughters, relatives or friends of influential people were appointed, resulting in a lack of support for CHWs by villagers and high drop-out rates (11).

Perhaps one of the most difficult aspects of representation arises when national politics are mixed with community development. In some countries the structure of the national government or ruling party extends down to the local level so that the community council is an organ of the national structure. Unless such bodies enjoy true popular support, there is a risk that health committees will represent only party interests and villagers may not even express opinions. It is not involvement of people secured under duress and obedience that should be the goal but their participation and cooperation (39).

The imposition of national interests on communities applies to bureaucracies as well as political structures. Ministries of health may engage in top-down planning whereby goals, objectives and priorities are determined in capital cities by professionals who have never lived in the communities that are the focus of their efforts. Goals may even be directed more by donor interests than by national interests. Because most national CHW programmes are characterized by top-down planning, with little involvement of local authorities, many villages are "littered with the carcasses of moribund committees and organizations" (15).

In some countries attempts have been made to ensure greater representation on committees. In the Gambia, village headmen and their councils are not representative of the population at large so the government specified that village development committees should include representatives of all major ethnic and caste groups in a defined area (40).

Efforts to decentralize health care have also contributed to more representative participation. In Sri Lanka, decentralization has resulted in the active participation of nongovernmental organizations and village-based governmental organizations in the activities of health teams at village level (41). In general decentralization efforts have been extended to the district health system but not yet to counties and villages. At district level participation has increased and, as this is institutionalized, greater community participation is expected.

Selecting health committee chairpersons and members

Not infrequently, the village leader or headman becomes the chairperson of the village health committee. Experience from the United Republic of Tanzania, among other places, indicates that the work of the committees suffers if these chairpersons are weak, uninterested or unpopular (30). Conversely, conscientious and motivated village leaders can make important contributions to health care programmes (39). In the Gambia, village development committees that are chaired by knowledgeable and active headmen perform well and are supported by the people. However, there have also been significant numbers of committees whose work was limited by a poor understanding of primary health care on the part of the chairpersons whose main interests were in providing drugs and curative care.

The leadership capacities of village health committee chairpersons and members are important ingredients for success. The orientation and training given to these persons are also important. Many programmes have failed to prepare committees to undertake their responsibilities (13). For example, lack of understanding of what primary health care services would be provided to villages by CHWs in the Sudan led to remarkable variation in the expectations of community leaders. Ninety-eight per cent thought that CHWs were to provide curative care, 65% thought they would have a preventive role, and only 30% understood there to be a role in health promotion (11).

Community leaders and members of health committees are expected to organize and manage community participation and health activities. This requires technical knowledge, an understanding of CHWs and primary health care, and skills in management and supervision. Skills training is not often provided to health committees. Committee members need to be able to carry out both simple tasks (electing leadership, conducting meetings) and complex ones (organizing communities, resolving conflict, administering funds). Several Kenyan programmes have provided training to village chiefs, assistant chiefs and committee members, as well as to specific target groups such as church leaders and school teachers (29). The training greatly enhanced committee support of CHWs.

These problems can be addressed through improved selection or replacement of committee leadership and through proper orientation and training. If a chairperson is a village headman but is weak, it may be possible to convince him to add a more able member of his council to the village health committee.

Improving the preparation and training of committees will require additional resources and improved communication. The process of introducing CHWs to the community, setting up the committee and creating expectations can be planned and evaluated. With appropriate personnel and response to constraints as they are encountered (rather than years later), a better committee can be built.

After committees are formed, they will still require practical training. This is probably best accomplished over time as they come together as a group and become more knowledgeable about the issues that they need to address. The resource and time requirements for this process of committee development should not be underestimated. It is reasonable to expect a process of months and years rather than of days or weeks.

Using community structures

In many primary health care and CHW programmes, participation structures and mechanisms are imposed on communities from the outside. In Kenya, a malaria control project established health committees covering 100 households in 36 villages. Committee members were selected on the basis of age, sex and social status. The committees were active only for short periods of time when they were engaged in specific activities and were not able to motivate villagers on a continuing basis. The project leaders concluded that it was inappropriate to reorganize the community for participation in health care or to set up a new leadership system of the village health committees. Instead, it was best to strengthen and work within the existing leadership and community organization structures, such as clans, women and other activity groups. The more peripheral to the community, the more ineffective village health committees were as a means of community involvement (42).

Where existing community organizations function well, it is far more effective to use them. Such organizations usually have a means for dialogue and discussion and enable the health programme to be incorporated into existing structures. Community organizations provide opportunities for lasting solutions to the problems of leadership, organization, resource mobilization and management (43).

The availability and effectiveness of local organizations vary. However, virtually all communities have organizations of some kind. CHW programmes are well advised to identify these organizations at the outset.

Involving community groups

Some CHW programmes work closely with special interest groups since these often have many members in the community. To improve health it is essential to involve as many human resources as possible, especially in preventive and promotive activities. The involvement of special interest groups can increase access to communities, promote intersectoral collaboration, and help to mobilize the will and resources to accomplish health-related tasks. In the context of primary health care and CHW programmes the most important special interest groups may be women's associations.

Women's associations

Women's associations are often involved in village health activities, although they are not necessarily represented on village health committees. Women are especially important because it is they who primarily take care of children, and children under the age of five are the most vulnerable group in any community. Women in their childbearing years are also far more likely to be in poor health or to die than men of the same age. Because of this, women and young children are often the focus of primary health care and CHW programmes. For socioeconomic and cultural reasons women are often much more difficult to reach with health services than men are. In some cases women's groups may be the only socially acceptable channel for doing this. Many women's groups are well organized and capable of planning, coordinating and implementing health activities. Some could provide the foundation for more comprehensive health programmes.

In the Saradidi rural health project in Kenya, women's associations were among the most important voluntary partners. Although they were not represented on the village health committees they informally took on some committee tasks. They provided more effective support to the CHWs than did the elected leadership (37). In the 1987 national vaccination campaigns in Senegal, women's organizations held local meetings to ensure that mothers brought their children to the vaccination posts (44). In Nepal, during the early stages of the female CHW programme, a national women's organization was designated an official partner to the Ministry of Health and assisted in the organization of mothers' groups and the recruitment and selection of community health volunteers (45).

Women's associations are more formally represented on village health committees in the Gambia and some other countries. Many of the representatives are the leaders of local women's organizations that undertake communal farming (40). In villages in north-western Somalia there is one woman for every four or five members of each village health committee. However, the role of women may vary considerably from village to village. In some, they are outspoken experts in maternal and child health, while in others they serve only to fulfil a requirement of the district health team (34).

Although women may have little visible authority, they are important to community health and represent an experienced resource for CHW programmes. Programmes that neglect to involve women will fail to reach the most vulnerable sector of the community.

Religious groups

Religious groups play an important role in health development in many countries. In addition to establishing comprehensive local health care projects, including CHW programmes, they provide assistance in many related areas. In Algeria, Senegal and Turkey, imams have taken an active role in urging parents to have their children vaccinated during national campaigns (46). In Myanmar, the CHW programme has sought the help of Buddhist monks (11). In Colombia, the Roman Catholic church has trained over 5000 parish agents to teach child survival techniques to parents in remote areas (47). Religious groups often work intensively in villages in poor and underserved areas (46). They provide practical examples of how communities can be enabled to manage and implement their own social services.

Schools, teachers and students

In many communities, schools carry out health projects and provide health training for specific groups. However, most of the health activities undertaken by schools are initiated by governmental organizations or NGOs, or are the work of a particularly motivated teacher. It is not clear to what extent schools and their teachers collaborate with CHWs or are involved systematically in primary health care. Nonetheless, since schools are valued by communities and since they educate the next generation, school involvement in community health care may be one of the most productive areas of intersectoral collaboration open to CHW programmes.

In Nepal, a rural development programme and a secondary school jointly implemented a health education and sanitation project in which students were taught about the need for latrines and learned how to build them. After returning to their home villages, the students motivated and assisted families to build simple latrines. The project was so successful that it was extended to other schools in the area. Health post staff, village leaders and respected community members also participated (48).

The idea of training schoolchildren to be health workers is gaining credibility. It is both practical and effective not only because children are future adults but because they often care for younger children at home. If taught enthusiastically, children can readily influence adults and can serve as resource persons within each household. In many homes in the

35

developing world, children attending school are the first generation to be literate. With appropriate support, schoolchildren can have a considerable impact on health knowledge and practice. This is especially so in the case of female students.

The range of roles that can be played by students and teachers is wide. In Bangladesh, schoolchildren have been trained to use oral rehydration therapy, while in the United Republic of Tanzania schoolteachers provide health education lessons to the community. Some schools assist health workers by taking part in screening programmes such as the one for schistosomiasis which is described in Box 8.

Farmers' groups, labour organizations and cooperatives

There is little documentation about the functions of these groups in health development. However, most rural populations are farmers, and many local farmers' associations exist. Their main activities relate to food production and marketing but they also deal with processes that have significant health effects such as water supply and irrigation. Given

---

BOX 8

Schools help screening for schistosomiasis

United Republic of Tanzania

The importance of schools and schoolteachers in health development has been recognized in the United Republic of Tanzania. In addition to providing health education to schoolchildren, teachers have also successfully participated in screening for urinary schistosomiasis.

In Kilosa District a large number of schools were invited to participate in the screening project. In the first stage some 15 000 primary schoolchildren were interviewed by their teachers over a four-week period using simple questionnaires. In the second stage, the head teachers of 49 high-risk and 26 low-risk schools carried out a test on 80 children using reagent sticks to detect haematuria. Within six weeks, 5750 children were screened. Cross-checks in 18 schools confirmed the accuracy of the head teachers' testing. This allowed the results to be used for the epidemiological mapping of the district and for the treatment of those children whose tests were positive.

This two-stage approach depended entirely on the existing school system. For only US$3000 a rural district of 15 000 km^2 and 350 000 inhabitants were screened within four months. This was twice as fast and eight times cheaper than screening with the standard urine filtration method. This approach means that district authorities do not have to depend entirely on specialized screening teams.

Source: Lengeler et al. (*49*).

---

the importance of nutrition and waterborne diseases, these associations seem likely targets for cooperation with primary health care and CHW programmes.

In the Philippines, one church-based health programme specifically sought the cooperation of the local farmers' organization. This group was experienced in organizing activities, overseeing them and mobilizing resources for them. Some of the activities were also important to the functioning of the health care services. The experience of the farmers' organization made an important contribution to the success of the programme (44). In many places, there are similar organizations for other kinds of rural workers that may be interested in health promotion. In Burkina Faso, for instance, such an organization has helped to develop self-help groups to further social and economic development at local level. These groups construct dams and dykes, anti-erosion works, and wells. They also manage rural pharmacies and primary health care services (50).

Other groups

In some countries Boy Scouts, Girl Guides and sports organizations have already taken part in immunization campaigns. Groups that have participated in community health programmes include school nutrition clubs, adult literacy teachers and rural shopkeepers. Often these groups served as the sole communications links with villages that might otherwise have been difficult to reach. Community organizations perform important functions for people's well-being and are a "hidden health promotion system" (32).

Lessons learned

The importance and potential benefit of active village health committees are not in question. In order to improve CHW programmes, these committees or other appropriate groups that represent communities need to be strengthened and expanded. Lessons learned from experience have been documented and it is possible to suggest some basic principles. Village health committees should:
- be representative of the entire local population to be served by the health programme;
- be chaired by highly motivated and capable persons who enjoy the support of the community;
- be based on existing leadership and organizational structures;
- include representatives from existing community organizations (if it is not possible to include representatives from all groups, others should be invited to send observers to committee meetings);

— have members who are adequately trained for their responsibilities.

The community and the CHW

Village health committees make decisions and carry out administrative tasks but the community members themselves are involved in a range of daily activities that have direct or indirect impact on health. The primary health care approach calls for community members who are not simply passive recipients of care but active participants in health development.

CHWs are in principle active community members who have accepted positions to promote good health and who serve as links between the community and the formal health system. Whether volunteers or salaried, their commitment to improving health is the same. The community cooperates with CHWs in return for services, and provides support as necessary. In the case of salaried workers this support may take the form of social assistance or extra help when there is a lot of work to do. In the case of volunteers the support may need to be more substantial. An active CHW volunteer has limited time to devote to earning money. The community and sometimes the health system compensate for the work in cash or in kind. However, remuneration of CHWs has been a major problem in many national programmes since the regularity and intensity of support differ from one place to another (*37*).

In the District of Ketou in Benin, the CHW programme was accepted with great enthusiasm. After initial sensitization, members of the community participated actively in the construction of latrines and carbon-based water filters. Communities continue to report that CHWs are important. However, they have not been able to remunerate CHWs out of the income from drug sales as planned and have not identified alternatives (*11*).

In the Saradidi programme in Kenya, villagers and CHWs work together frequently. CHWs have regular contact with village elders and with women's groups. Community members take part in health activities as and when they are able: men donate money for projects, children carry messages, and women organize groups to clean villages. This active involvement appears to be a result of efforts to sensitize the whole population and to build on the established Anglican church to which one-third of the inhabitants belong. Initially, the congregation set up committees to talk to other congregations and to village leaders about the benefits of a community health programme. Other members approached individuals and families in their own neighbourhoods. Within three months most people in the community were aware of the programme and their own potential roles in it. The fact that the programme was initiated by the community itself and not by outsiders appears to have made it easier to get people involved (*11*).

In many other CHW programmes the links between the population and the CHW are more distant and do not function well. Studies have identified several factors that have a negative effect on the relationship between communities and CHWs.

- Many communities do not have full confidence in CHWs because community members are neither adequately informed nor consulted during the selection process. In Zimbabwe almost all CHWs said they had been selected by communities though interviews revealed this was true in only one-third of the cases (51).
- In some programmes the CHWs are employed by the government and placed in health clinics where they assist nursing staff. Contact with the community is limited to outpatient visits and occasional home visits. CHWs do not have the opportunity to build and maintain close links with individuals and families in villages.
- In some communities CHWs are not valued because they cannot meet expectations for curative care. People suffering from common health problems usually want treatment and are not satisfied with health education and advice (52). Chronic shortages of drugs in most CHW programmes also contribute to community dissatisfaction. Unless health promotive activities are provided in conjunction with adequate treatment for common diseases the credibility of CHWs is likely to decline.
- The reluctance or inability of many communities to support CHWs with resources also diminishes their relationship. The problems of lack of support have been documented frequently and most often reflect unwillingness to pay CHWs for benefits that are considered small (53). Very poor communities may not be able to find the money needed to remunerate CHWs. At the same time, CHWs who are not compensated for their work may not be able to devote much time to volunteer activities. A gain in status is inadequate motivation for many CHWs who are sole providers for their families (54).
- CHWs often do not have the skills or ability to communicate with and mobilize the community well. These skills are not emphasized in training sessions and supervisors may be ill-prepared to provide them. Consequently the quality of the community-CHW interaction depends on the capabilities of individuals.
- In many instances communities are not adequately sensitized to the benefits of CHW programmes, and are not aware of the role of the CHW or the importance of community participation. CHWs themselves have not always been properly trained and some do not have a clear understanding of what they are expected to do for the community (55). Misperceptions and wrong expectations on the part of both the community and the CHW can undermine their relationship.

39

Intensive efforts are required to establish and nurture a working partnership between CHWs and communities. Small-scale community health projects managed by NGOs have been more successful in developing this partnership, but they also often build on years of experience working in the same locations. In order to establish a partnership between CHWs and communities in the context of health development some basic principles must be followed:

* Sufficient numbers of community members must understand the primary health care approach, the need for community participation, and the role of CHWs. Similarly, CHWs must be both trained and enabled to work in partnership with communities.
* CHWs must be selected through a representational process that involves many, if not all, community members. This will lay the foundation for respect and confidence in providing primary health care.
* CHWs are responsible for supporting the health development of all families in their villages or communities. This responsibility cannot be assumed properly by CHWs who spend most of their time in health centres.
* CHWs should be adequately equipped to respond to the most urgent needs of the community, including the provision of basic curative care when no other health services are readily available.
* Effective means of supporting or compensating CHWs must be found in order to ensure their sustainability. CHWs, like other villagers, must secure the livelihood of their families.

Involving traditional healers

Working partnerships between the formal health care system and traditional healers vary with national or local circumstances. Such a partnership is more common where political support for the place of traditional medicine is found at national level, as in China and India. Elsewhere traditional medicine is often not strongly represented in CHW programmes. The integration of modern and traditional medical systems is often talked of in general terms as a guiding principle for CHW programmes but it is important to examine what this means in practice.

Modern medicine is made available to people through an identifiable organizational structure which people can see and which, in most respects, is outside their own social network. Indigenous medicine is usually quite different. People have various choices, including the services of specialist healers, but where major traditions such as Ayurvedic medicine are not prominent there is generally no overall medical system or structure.

While integration between the formal health care sector and traditional medicine may be difficult to achieve in some areas, it is important to remember that the user may view the two approaches as complementary and may see no conflict between them. It is normal in most countries for people to use the various options that are open to them. This implies that CHW programmes must attempt to relate constructively to other prevailing systems of healing.

If CHW programmes forge links and avoid conflicts with traditional providers of care, the programmes will build confidence and support for their own activities.

The term "traditional healer" usually refers to one or more of the following: herbalist, diviner, spiritual or faith healer, traditional midwife, traditional birth attendant, curandero, shaman, traditional Chinese doctor, Ayurvedic doctor, or Unani practitioner (56). Although they usually do not constitute an organized interest group, traditional medical practitioners are important providers of primary health care in the community.

Traditional healers are often highly respected in villages and community members have confidence in their opinions and advice.

In 1990–1991, WHO conducted a worldwide survey of projects where traditional healers were trained and functioned as CHWs (56). These projects were located in Africa, the Americas, Eastern Mediterranean, the Pacific and South-East Asia. Most were government-sponsored, though two were sponsored by NGOs.

Literature reviews, narrative descriptions, and views of experts in the field provided additional insight and suggestions as to how traditional healers can promote primary health care in communities. All this information has been reviewed and shows that there are a number of positive aspects to the use of traditional healers as CHWs.

Advantages of using traditional healers as CHWs

Traditional healers are willing to work in community health care.

The data supports the conclusion that traditional healers are willing to take on primary health care activities when they are given training and can establish good working relations with existing health staff. To date, a variety of healers have been trained to work in primary health care projects in a wide range of cultures.

Eight of the 17 projects surveyed by WHO have trained either traditional birth attendants or village midwives. Other projects have trained herbalists and spiritual healers in Africa and Latin America, Ayurvedic and Unani practitioners in India, traditional healers in Nepal, and bonesetters and magico-religious practitioners in Latin America. In each case, traditional healers were willing and available to undergo training and were enthusiastic in accepting their new roles in primary health care.

41

Traditional healers can be trained to perform a wide range of primary health care tasks.

The study indicated that it is possible to train traditional healers in a wide range of primary health care tasks. The projects trained healers for a variety of tasks, but all were related to one or more of the elements of primary health care. The following is a summary of skills taught to traditional healers, based on the eight elements of primary health care.

- Promoting education concerning prevailing health problems and the methods of preventing and controlling them, including:
  — giving information about local health problems;
  — demonstrating methods of preventing and controlling these problems;
  — using posters and other simple health education materials.

- Promoting improved food supply and proper nutrition, including:
  — showing how to obtain a balanced diet;
  — encouraging a proper diet for mother and child (i.e. breastfeeding and proper weaning foods);
  — growing vegetables and fruit in kitchen gardens.

- Promoting adequate supply of safe water and basic sanitation, including:
  — how to obtain safe water;
  — how to construct and use latrines properly;
  — how to maintain personal hygiene and sanitation in the home;
  — how to prepare and store food hygienically.

- Promoting maternal and child health care, including:
  — monitoring pregnancy and recognizing abnormalities;
  — giving proper antenatal care;
  — providing basic delivery techniques;
  — identifying when to refer women for abnormal conditions of delivery;
  — advising women about family planning;
  — distributing oral contraceptives and providing referral for other contraceptive methods.

- Promoting immunization against the major infectious diseases, including:
  — explaining when and how to refer children under five to clinics for immunization against childhood diseases.

- Promoting prevention and control of locally endemic diseases, including:
  — recognizing symptoms of dangerous conditions such as diarrhoea,

tuberculosis, leprosy, malaria and malnutrition and referring for treatment;
— demonstrating how to mix and use oral rehydration salts to treat dehydration and diarrhoea;
— distributing packets of oral rehydration salts;
— referring women in high risk groups for treatment;
— using readily available allopathic medicines, (i.e. anti-malarial prophylaxis, oral rehydration therapy, etc.).

- Providing appropriate treatment of common diseases and injuries, including:
  — giving first aid;
  — preventing accidents.

- Providing essential drugs, including:
  — supplying aspirin and other first aid medications;
  — operating basic dispensaries.

Training traditional healers has produced several positive results.

Projects that have attempted to evaluate the results of training have reported a number of positive outcomes.

- Projects in Brazil, Ghana, Nepal, Sudan and Swaziland indicated that participants had a high degree of interest in and enthusiasm for learning new information and skills relating to primary health care.
  These same projects were able to demonstrate changes in the practices of traditional healers after the training workshops. These changes included the following:
  — increased use of oral rehydration salts and giving of fluids to children with diarrhoea;
  — use of washbasins for washing hands in traditional healing clinics;
  — decreased use of strong purges and enemas for treating diarrhoea;
  — construction and use of latrines in traditional healers' homes;
  — increased referrals to clinics for patients with dangerous symptoms;
  — increase in the number of births attended by village midwives.

- While few data were reported on changes in health status of target populations, a number of projects indicated a high degree of acceptance by communities of the healers who had been trained. The project in Sudan reported that the proportion of women aged 30–34 years using contraceptives increased from 25% to 38% over the two-year period, and that overall use of contraceptives rose from 13% to 21%. The project in Nepal reported an increased attendance at rural clinics after trained traditional healers began working in local communities.

- Many of the projects indicated that there was an increase in trust and respect between the nursing staff and trained traditional healers, and that working relationships between the two groups improved. The project in Swaziland reported that there was an increase in referrals by traditional healers to rural clinics, particularly for children with diarrhoea and vomiting.

- Evaluation of the *dhami jhankri* (traditional healer) training programme in Nepal found conclusive evidence that faith healers can play a culturally appropriate and cost-effective role in health education and family planning. The staff estimated that countrywide there was a ratio of well over 100 *dhami jhankries* to each health worker and that these healers, as private practitioners, were paid only a modest fee for their services.

    In Swaziland, the cost to the government for materials and training of traditional healers in primary health care was relatively low. The government does not pay for services provided by traditional healers since they are private practitioners and are paid by the community. The Swaziland Traditional Healers Organization committed a large amount of time and resources to the project, which helped reduce the cost to the government.

    In the Philippines, project staff felt the main strength of the community-based health programme was its low cost. This was due to the project's employing traditional medical practitioners who used low-cost traditional therapies. Using traditional remedies that were locally available rather than commercially prepared drugs reduced costs.

Constraints on using traditional healers as CHWs

The training and use of traditional healers in community health worker programmes can pose difficulties in some situations.

For instance, positive government policies to promote cooperation and use of traditional healers in primary health care are often lacking. Lack of government commitment in some projects has discouraged healers from coming forward to participate in programmes designed to train them in primary health care skills. In those countries which have, until recently, prohibited traditional healers from practising, many healers are reluctant to participate in government-sponsored health programmes. The absence of government policies that acknowledge the positive role traditional healers can play has tended to reinforce secrecy about traditional healing practices in many countries.

There is also often a lack a dialogue between traditional healers and government health staff. This creates misunderstanding between the two groups and has prevented open and creative discussions to identify common health goals and ways of cooperating in providing better health care.

Some traditional practices, of course, may be harmful and difficult to change. Some practices can cause dangerous psychological stress and even bodily harm. Because of these and other factors, there often exists a conflict between traditional and modern medical practice. Even where traditional healing practices do not cause harm, the contrast between the traditional holistic, spiritual healing orientation and the modern biomedical treatment-oriented approach reveals a basic difference in philosophy regarding the causation of disease and the promotion of health. Differences in orientation and training can cause barriers between traditional and modern practitioners that prevent them from working in cooperation, but these barriers are not insurmountable where there is mutual respect and communication.

Charlatans and fraudulent practitioners obscure the worthwhile contributions of the majority of bona fide traditional healers. Isolated incidents of witchcraft, malpractice or unscrupulous behaviour are widely publicized by the media and tend to reinforce the stereotype of traditional healers as quacks. The fraudulent practice of a few inhibits better understanding and cooperation between the traditional and modern health sectors.

Lack of community participation in both the planning and implementation of primary health care projects where traditional healers are used has also caused difficulties. Given that the ultimate purpose of primary health care programmes is to improve community health, it is imperative that communities be represented in the selection and training of traditional healers who are designated to work in primary health care.

The fact that many traditional healers lack formal education and have low levels of literacy can pose difficulties for their training. In CHW projects in both Ghana and Swaziland, it was found that the poor literacy and education of some traditional healers required special training methods. Conventional methods such as lectures and use of written materials were not appropriate.

When the role of the traditional healer in relation to other members of the primary health care team is not clearly defined, and the tasks to be performed are not specifically described, problems have arisen. In Nigeria, because the role of the traditional healers was not made clear, some feared that their integration in the primary health care programme might threaten their status, income and freedom of action in the community.

Lack of cooperation impairs coordination of services between traditional healers and health staff. One example of this is the difficulty of establishing referral systems between traditional healers and clinic staff.

Box 9 describes how traditional healers in Botswana agreed to refer patients with certain symptoms following a training workshop.

Links between the health system and the health development structure

Links between the health system and the health development structure are often informal and specific to particular communities. They may be influenced by politics and economics, by the social distance between health workers and communities, and by community beliefs and attitudes to care-seeking. Further, what is needed to develop these links may differ at district and local levels.

If CHWs can be considered one of the links between the community and the formal health system, then the attitudes and behaviours of the health system toward the health development structure may be seen partly in the level of support and encouragement it provides to CHWs. For many national and district health systems, CHW programmes are low priority. Clinic-based curative care and focused disease control programmes often occupy most health workers, despite the fact that health services alone will not contribute much to the prevention of ill-health and death in the communities. This is reflected in limited interactions with CHWs and the allocation of insufficient resources to enable CHWs to carry out their tasks either as service providers or as agents of change. Since the attitudes of health workers towards CHWs are often negative and there is little understanding of or belief in their importance to the health system and to improved health, it is not difficult to

---

BOX 9

Traditional practitioners participate in health development

Botswana

At a health seminar for community leaders, the participants suggested that there was a need for communication and cooperation between traditional healers and modern health workers. The community leaders felt that coordination of the two health care systems would improve people's health. A joint workshop was held for traditional practitioners, faith healers and modern health workers, as a result of which the traditional healers accepted certain principles of modern medicine—such as the use of oral rehydration salts for the treatment of diarrhoea—and agreed to promote them.

They also agreed, as a matter of course, to refer patients with symptoms suggestive of tuberculosis or with bleeding in pregnancy. Some traditional health practitioners are members of village health committees, which promotes the exchange of information.

Source: Health for all: from words to deeds (*57*).

---

see that health workers may not recognize or value other parts of a community's health development structure.

Several factors influence community involvement in health and the nature of links with the health system. These factors include political commitment to the idea of people's involvement, the extent to which authority is decentralized and community involvement is possible, the economic situation and the allocation of resources to social sectors, and the level of development of local structures and organizations (*11*). The extent to which links can be developed and at what speed will depend on these environmental factors. For example, in Zimbabwe the speed of development of democratic institutions in society dictated the pace and success of community involvement with village health workers. An example of successful community sensitization and involvement in Venezuela is given in Box 10.

There are very few functional links between the health system and local organizations involved in health development (*58*). Those that exist have been established in response to specific situations and may not

---

BOX 10

Community sensitization provides tangible results

Venezuela

In a project for the control of Chagas disease in Venezuela, it was found that when community members were properly sensitized to a programme, agreed to its usefulness and understood their own responsibilities within it, their participation contributed greatly to its success.

Traditionally, Chagas disease has been controlled by spraying houses with residual insecticides in order to kill the triatomine bug that transmits it. However, problems with this method prompted the testing of a new approach by the social studies department of the Central University of Venezuela and the housing department of the State of Cojedes.

The project produced designs for house construction which were acceptable to communities, which could be built by the people themselves, and which resulted in environments unfavourable to the Chagas disease vector. The techniques and materials used were familiar and affordable. Participation in the project was voluntary, but rules were established from the start. People received technical assistance but were responsible for constructing their own houses. Loans were made available but had to be repaid in full.

The new houses proved to be free of triatomine bugs. They were also highly valued by the people who had committed themselves to building them. Functional and valued links between government services and communities had been established and were continued. As a result of the project, the Ministry of Health revised its policies for controlling Chagas disease. Funds allocated to insecticide spraying were redirected to improved housing.

Source: Briceno-Leon (*59*).

---

last long. For example, as a result of programme evaluations, efforts to strengthen CHW programmes have been directed at increasing community participation. To do this, local organizations involved in health development are identified and analysed and health workers are encouraged to make them more active. In the case of village health committees this should involve reorientation, education, negotiation, and perhaps the decentralization of decision-making in areas such as drug supply or the planning of CHW workloads. In practice, health workers are not provided with guidance on how to accomplish increased activity and efforts to achieve improvement may be limited to attending a few meetings and lecturing those present on what they should be doing. This is not likely to result in truly functional links that can be expanded over time for other purposes. It is more likely to result in frustration on the part of health workers and community members.

There have been some attempts to address these problems, as in the Zimbabwe CHW programme. The problem of poor community support, as reflected in lack of remuneration of CHWs and poor orientation to CHW roles, was addressed by working with local authorities to ensure that CHWs were paid, by starting projects that could give seed money to pay CHWs and by providing in-service training to CHWs to develop skills in community involvement, health education, communication and the use of a management information system.

The problems associated with interactions between health workers and CHWs have been discussed earlier. They result in conflicting attitudes and relationships that hinder the development of working partnerships. They are the result of poor supervision and communication, lack of understanding of community-based primary health care, unrealistic expectations, lack of clear vision and goals, and insufficient resources. These issues need to be addressed in order to improve links with the health development structure and broaden the range of resources available to CHW activities.

A call for action

The people and organizations that form the health development structure are important potential contributors to the improvement of health in communities. They can complement the district health system.

A number of efforts can be made within the context of CHW programmes to develop the links between the health development structure and the district health system. These efforts involve:

— allocation of resources and orientation and sensitization of communities prior to the initiation of programmes;
— within existing programmes, reorientation and negotiation with communities about participation in programme activities;

— activation of village health committees or other appropriate groups as decision-makers for programmes, including re-evaluation of roles and responsibilities, and efforts to increase meaningful participation (training in management and communication skills may be necessary);

— review and expansion of social mobilization for health projects (with the emphasis on ongoing support);

— re-evaluation of CHW roles and tasks, and negotiation with communities regarding what they expect, what can be achieved within the constraints of resources and what is desirable for public health (advocacy for vulnerable groups and education about community health problems may be necessary);

— improvement of the attitudes of health workers and CHWs towards community health and each other, within the context of strengthening the district health system;

— development of CHWs as a group within the health development structure, able to form networks between and within communities to learn from each other and to assist each other;

— training of health workers and CHWs to recognize potential inputs from the health development structure (including the development of communication and negotiation skills, and the ability to manage joint activities);

— further study of health development structures and their potential contribution to the sustainability of CHW programmes.

Experience with NGOs and with global programmes such as those for immunization and community development shows that the health development structure is an underutilized resource that could enhance achievements and resolve problems of CHW programmes. Exactly how to utilize it more and nurture it may not be so clear, however. Local organizations and interest groups are formed for specific social reasons and purposes, and interesting them in the goals and activities of community health must be an effort of collaboration rather than cooption. Increasing the functional links between the health system and the health development structure may also require a better understanding of sustainability itself.

CHAPTER 3

Resources

The Alma-Ata Conference in 1978 was followed by greatly expanded political commitment to providing primary health care, with governments trying out new ways of increasing the availability of care at reasonable cost. CHWs had been successful in performing basic health care tasks in small-scale projects, and it seemed feasible to expand the concept to national programmes. It was thought that these programmes would alleviate immediate needs for access to health care, would extend the current reach of government resources, and would be affordable. Affordable essentially meant that recurrent costs to government health systems would be low. Financing would be made possible, it was anticipated, through donor funding of high initial investment costs, with the subsequent recurrent costs shared between governments and communities.

As CHW programmes were expanded in different countries, the increased costs of this expansion became apparent. While it was possible for local programmes to have low unit costs and to be efficient, programmes aimed at large populations and with wide geographic scope generated high overall costs. In addition, many costs were hidden and assumed to be absorbed by the health system as CHW programmes were grafted onto existing primary health care services. Programmes were introduced with varying combinations of government, community and fee-for-service support, but weaknesses in this ad hoc approach quickly arose. These included problems with the remuneration of CHWs, deficiencies in the support services required for effective CHW functioning, poor planning and inadequate budgeting which created unrealistic expectations, and underestimation of how to build enough community involvement to generate contributions in kind or in cash. Government decision-makers, donors and communities alike became disillusioned. The question of sustainability, closely associated with financing, was brought to the forefront. After all, political commitment to primary health care, even after Alma-Ata, was often not matched by financial commitent.

To allocate resources more realistically, policy-makers require sound information. Countries should identify all the essential elements of their CHW programmes, make the necessary cost estimates, identify financial resources, and communicate the information effectively in order to obtain adequate budgetary allocations. Planning for financing will require clear decisions about CHW roles and responsibilities with regard to curative, preventive and promotive services.

Providing resources to CHWs is an investment in the capacity of the health care system. CHWs can participate effectively in both "vertical" disease-specific programmes and in primary health care. As decentralization and community involvement in health increases, it will become clear that CHWs are not an alternative programme but are an integral part of a long-term strategy to improve public health. The documented effectiveness of CHWs in the areas of prevention and promotion, and their utility in situations with different levels of economic development, should make it clear that they are not simply a solution for the poor. CHW programmes have progressed a long way from the time they were considered stop-gap measures and have demonstrated their potential to improve health.

General concerns

CHW programmes have increased both the coverage and equity of primary health care services at low cost compared to other service delivery strategies (11). However, the total amount of resources needed to provide CHW programmes nationally is large. In addition to high initial investment costs, the programmes need substantial reinvestment in training, management, logistics and supervision (6). It is important to note, however, that although the resource needs of well-supported CHW programmes are higher than the limited resources usually made available they are only a small proportion of total national health expenditure or even total government expenditure on health. As a result of resource constraints in many developing countries during the past decade, the health sector has experienced real declines in financing, and expenditures for curative and higher level health care have been better protected than those for primary and preventive care. CHW programmes, as the most peripheral part of health systems, have been particularly affected. Inadequate and declining resources have also led to questions about issues such as the remuneration of CHWs, support services required for effective CHW functioning, planning and budgeting, and the need for effective community contributions.

Remuneration of CHWs

The WHO Study Group on Community Health Workers reaffirmed the necessity of remunerating CHWs if the time required to carry out the functions assigned is a significant proportion of the day.

Decisions on whether, or how much, CHWs should be paid, and who should pay depend upon the type of function they are expected to perform. These matters cannot be prescribed. Governments must define what type of CHW programme the country needs, and what priority and resources it is prepared to allocate to it vis-à-vis other needs. This will determine whether funds are available to finance the programme, including the payment of CHWs. If governments continue to allocate a high proportion of their health budgets to tertiary health care, and to medical services and personnel, it is unlikely that they will have the resources to cover adequately the costs of preventive and other primary health care services, let alone to provide incentives for CHWs or pay their wages . . .

There is no one definitive answer to the question of who should pay CHWs. It is determined mainly by the type of programme. If it is highly structured, and the CHW has specific responsibilities and is accountable to an authority for the performance of a set of tasks, then it is normal for the authority, whether government, nongovernmental organization or local council, to pay. However, a CHW who is accountable mainly to the community, or performs only services that are required by the community, can be expected to charge the community for services in cash or in kind, or the community may decide on a suitable recompense. The Study Group warned against a "fee-for-service" arrangement, because of the tendency it induces in CHWs to concentrate on curative services, for which they can charge fees, and thereby to neglect preventive and health promotional tasks (2).

Support services

The range of support services required for effective CHW functioning includes training, supervision, personnel management, logistics and supply, monitoring and evaluation. It is now clear that it cannot simply be assumed that the existing infrastructure will take on these tasks without guidance and support. The support needed can take either financial or other forms, such as the increasing recognition of activities performed with CHWs. Support needs to be planned and costed, and the results used to convince health planners and policy-makers of the need to provide it.

Planning and budgeting for CHW programmes

Lack of information and understanding of true programme costs contributes to the lack of resources and the unrealistic expectations of what CHWs can do. In the short term these cause frustration and dissatisfaction, while in the long term they undermine the peripheral health system.

The lack of adequate budgeting for CHW programmes is often associated with the absence of defined cost items, which leads to unrealistic plans. Governments have sometimes also been misled into thinking that a shift of emphasis from institutional to community services will result in expanding services at no cost to government. Experience now shows, however, that the costs of training, supervision, personnel and transport can be very high, and that these items require careful planning and make considerable demands on government expenditure (2).

Requirements for effective community involvement and contribution

It is commonly assumed that community involvement entails no more than contributing to a programme in cash or in kind. It implies much more, however, including participation in programme planning from its inception, and in its financial management. Communities must be guided in understanding their role and what they should expect from the CHW programme (2).

As primary health care services are decentralized and increasing community participation is expected, the need to understand and balance community involvement in health with government and NGO support will become more critical.

It is a general view that communities should contribute towards the costs of CHW programmes. This increases self-reliance and may be a key to community participation. However, since many communities cannot afford the total cost, the deficiency has to be made good by the government and by nongovernmental organizations. On no account, however, should the community be subjected to "double taxation": supporting both the formal health system, including the sophisticated urban services, and its own CHW programme (2).

Costs of CHWs

CHWs have been classed as programmes in much the same way as disease control interventions such as the Expanded Programme on Immunization (EPI) or Control of Diarrhoeal Diseases (CDD). Yet CHWs are available to the community usually for a variety of health-related tasks. Disease control programmes are often vertical and have separate

53

budgets, while CHW programmes are more horizontal with varying responsibilities to different budgeting authorities. In this context, the financial implications of properly supported national CHW programmes have not been determined. Some are funded entirely by governments, some entirely by communities, and sometimes the costs are shared by government, communities, voluntary organizations and external sources. However, it has proved difficult to sustain CHW programmes in times of economic difficulty when resources allocated to such programmes may be the first to be cut.

Although the cost of items such as training, CHW remuneration and supplies is generally known and to varying extents provided for, major elements such as the large amount of health personnel time and health services resources needed to support CHW programmes are neither known nor included in budgets. The failure to make cost assessments of this sort and to incorporate them in planning and delivery of health services has led to inadequate support of CHWs and neglect of activities, particularly for prevention.

It has been observed that one reason why there are many successful pilot projects but few examples of successful replication is that programmes are too dependent on external inputs. Donor inputs into community-based health care programmes usually make up a high proportion of the total budget for the initiation of programme activities. Frequently, the exact cost of running programmes is not known because various contributions or donations are not included in specific programme costs but remain as hidden subsidies (58).

Lack of information on hidden or poorly understood costs appears to be common. In its publication *Better health in Africa*, the World Bank does not put a cost on CHW programmes despite the fact they are recommended as an appropriate and cost-effective strategy for health service delivery in the African context (4). Given this situation, WHO has undertaken two case studies to determine the costs of CHW programmes in Jamaica and in Thailand.

Assessing the costs of CHW programmes in Thailand and Jamaica

To help governments estimate the costs of establishing and running CHW programmes, WHO conducted a series of field studies in various countries. These studies analyse the types and quantities of inputs required, as well as their costs, to help establish baseline data for national and international comparisons. Particular emphasis was put on the development of a methodological approach that could be readily used by health planners for cost analysis.

The two first studies were carried out in Jamaica and Thailand, where the governments had long experience in financing CHW programmes.

In Thailand, the first government-supported CHWs were introduced in 1964 and by 1986 the whole population had access to local CHWs. The Jamaican government initiated CHW programmes early and they have been available nationwide since 1972. In Thailand the study was undertaken in five villages in Lamphun Province, a rural area in the northern part of the country. In Jamaica three health districts in the parish of Hanover, Cornwall Country Health Region, were selected for investigation.

The CHW programmes in Thailand and Jamaica

In Thailand the CHW programme is an extension of the formal health system at village level. The role of the government is limited to providing general guidelines and support, while community involvement and self-reliance are basic principles for all local activities. The two main types of CHWs are the village health volunteers and the village health communicators.

The 70 000 village health volunteers undertake a range of primary health care activities, while the 600 000 village health communicators (one per 10–15 households) are primarily educators and promoters. The CHWs are supervised by the local health centres. They are members of the community and are closely involved with community development groups. They are not paid but receive free medical care as compensation for their work.

The CHW programme in Jamaica differs from that in Thailand. The Jamaican community health aides are paid health workers who extend health centre services to the villages. They spend half of their time on clinic-based work and half on field activities, including home visits. Although many community health aides are civil servants, they do not enjoy all the benefits normally received by government employees. In the Hanover parish only one-third of the community health aides trained originally were still active in 1989. Seventeen per cent had retired or emigrated while another 50% were laid off in 1985 and 1986 for economic reasons. The ratio of community health aides to number of population is now 1:2500, though regional distribution is uneven, ranging from 1:576 to 1:4206.

Methodological approach

It is possible to identify the various components or units of CHW programmes and estimate approximate costs in those areas. For example, the amount of time and its monetary value spent by administrators and health staff on various CHW related activities can be assessed. The costs of supplies, equipment and transport are somewhat easier to establish, although it may be necessary to estimate how these items are distributed among various health workers. The approximate total cost of the programme can be obtained by adding the costs of the different units. It is also necessary to take into account the support activities for CHWs at all levels of the health system.

However, when basing calculations of future costs on previous budgets, it is important to distinguish between budgeted and realized expenditures. Budgeted expenditures are estimates of financial provisions, while realized expenditures are the actual expenditures made. In many countries there are substantial differences between budgeted and realized expenditures. Therefore, the use of budgeted expenditures or realized expenditures alone may result in misleading cost estimates. For example, a health programme may receive a budget allocation of US$ 1000 for drugs but may spend only US$ 600 (60%). It is important to take into account whether the lower expenditure stems from a temporary shortage of drugs, or whether the original allocation was unnecessarily high. Underspending may represent an overestimated need and overspending an underestimated need, but there could also be financial problems. With regard to CHW programmes there is a notable discrepancy between pre-established supervisory schemes and the actual time health personnel spend on supervision. Care must be taken that adequate budget allocations are made for supervision, and that such allocations are not merely based on previous inadequate practices.

Categories of cost

There are two categories of cost that have to be taken into account.

- Investment costs are those incurred in establishing CHW programmes. They relate to initial planning and administration, recruitment and training of CHWs, training of CHW trainers, reorientation courses for health staff, and equipment, materials and vehicles used at this initial stage. They may also include the cost of mobilization of communities and training of community leaders.
- Recurrent or operational costs are the costs involved in running CHW programmes. These costs cover supervision, in-service training, drugs, equipment, materials, transport and general administration. If the CHWs are compensated (in Thailand they receive free health care), recurrent costs also include the remuneration or the estimated value of this compensation.

Programme costs are either direct or indirect.

- Direct costs usually correspond to local inputs such as supplies used by the CHWs and, in some countries, their remuneration.

56

- Indirect costs relate to the support provided to the CHW programme from other parts of the health system through administration, training, supervision and supplies. These costs are calculated as proportions of the overall resources used at these different levels, such as the proportion of district health worker salaries that corresponds to the time they spend supervising CHWs.

Data collection and sources of information

In Jamaica and Thailand, cost data were collected at national, provincial, district and local levels using information on budget and health service expenditure.

- At national level, extensive discussions on cost-related issues were held with various departments in the Ministry of Health, and particularly with the department responsible for primary health care. In addition, the unit costs for various services and activities were collected from Ministry of Health documentation. Information was also gathered on the resources used in different departments for training, production and distribution of educational materials, and for research directly related to CHW programmes. In Jamaica, background information on the community health aides programme was also obtained from the Department of Social and Preventive Medicine of the University of the West Indies.
- At provincial and district levels, information on the activities of CHWs was collected through structured interviews with health officials, including nursing and administrative staff.
- At local level in Thailand, interviews were conducted with CHWs and members of village health or development committees. Group discussions were used to establish the amount of time given and activities performed by health volunteers during the previous month.

In general CHWs do not keep activity or financial records. Therefore estimates had to be made on the basis of information collected in interviews. In Jamaica, interviews were held with community health aides and their supervisors at the health centre. The records of home visits made by 50% of the aides during the previous six months were also analysed.

Calculation of unit costs

When calculating the costs of the different components of CHW programmes, it is important to ensure that relevant subcomponents are included. Just which subcomponents should be taken into account will depend partly on the country concerned. In Jamaica, where unit costs were taken primarily from data and cost calculations available in the

Ministry of Health, terms had to be defined and subcomponents item-
ized. For example, the category "salaries" for personnel at national level
included basic salaries and allowances such as market premiums, uni-
form and motor vehicle maintenance. A fixed amount for health care
benefits (free hospital services for government employees) was based on
the assumption of a 10% probability of a 10-day hospital stay per year.
The category "transport and travel" included costs for vehicle operation,
drivers' salaries, public transport, and subsistence payments.

When calculating indirect costs, it is important to make accurate
estimates of the proportion of the overall resources at different levels of
the health system that are used for the CHW programme. At national
level in Jamaica the investment costs for planning and management
were, in addition to the employment of a full-time programme coordina-
tor for one year, estimated at two staff months for curriculum development. Travel costs were estimated at 10 field days with 200 miles of
vehicle use each day during the initial year. Unless the relevant subcomponents and their actual cost are included in calculations, there is a risk
that the costs of CHW programmes will be underestimated.

Costs of the CHW programme in Thailand[1]

In Thailand, 13% of the total government expenditure on health in
1990 was spent on the village health volunteer programme. The provincial health administrations, Provincial Chief Medical Offices
(PCMOs), receive an annual primary health care budget to develop and
run the CHW programme in their areas. In Lamphun Province,
this budget has been 5% of the total provincial health budget. It is the
largest of a number of programme budgets (such as family planning,
nutrition, environmental sanitation, and AIDS control) managed by the
PCMO.

In 1990, the Ministry of Public Health spent the equivalent of
US$ 476 580 on support to the village health volunteer programme in
Lamphun Province; 15.5% of this covered investment costs and 84.3%
covered operating costs. This corresponds to an average cost of
US$ 1930 per village. The Ministry contributed 17% of the investment
costs and 6% of the recurrent costs. The PCMO generated 34% of
the investment costs and 53% of the recurrent costs, while 43% of
the investment costs and 37% of the running costs were attributed to the
health centre level. The villages themselves also contributed to the
programme, essentially through the sale of drugs. In 1990, their contribution amounted to 25–49% of the government expenditure.

---

[1] The information presented in this section is based on the report of a study undertaken
by Dr Wolfgang Weber, University of Heidelberg, Germany, on the costs and financing
of health volunteer programmes in Lamphun Province, Thailand.

The primary health care budget of the PCMO mainly covers recruit-ment and training of new CHWs. Initial activities include census and mapping at the health centre level to collect basic demographic data on communities, and visits to villages to promote the CHW programme. Training covers training of trainers (travel costs and subsistence allowance), distribution of training materials, and initial training of CHWs.

Once the CHWs start working in the community their activities are supported by various levels of the health system.

• Management and planning of the CHW programme take place at all levels: central, provincial (PCMO), district (7 district health offices) and *tambon* (60 health centres). For the PCMO, these activities prima-rily involve budget development processes and financial control. As it is not possible to separate the management and planning activities related to the CHW programme from other management and plan-ning activities, it has been assumed that the proportion of resources used at this level (staff time and use of equipment) is roughly equal to the proportion of the total provincial health budget that is devoted to primary health care (i.e. 5%). In staff time, this corresponds to 80 days per year. In each of the seven district health offices (DHOs), the staff spend about 1.5% of their time, or three staff days per year, on village visits to monitor the programme, to identify needs to expand the programme and to replace CHWs. The *tambon* health centres are involved in the current administration of the CHW programme. In addition to keeping lists of CHWs, issuing CHW licences and coordinating programme activities, they organize monthly and yearly health worker meetings to monitor the programme and to plan activities. The health centre staff spend about half a day each month in health worker meetings and two further days in yearly meetings; this corresponds to 1.75% of their work time or about seven days per year.

• Most of the regular supervision of CHWs is carried out by the *tambon* health centre staff. Every village health post is visited once a month by a supervisor from the nearest health centre. An average of 12% of staff time, or four person days per month, is spent on such visits. The DHOs are also involved in the supervision of CHWs, although to a lesser degree. The DHOs are primarily responsible for supervising the health centres. DHO staff spend about 40 days per year on health centre visits, and one-third of this time—13.3 staff days or some 7% of their total time—is devoted to CHW-related issues. Moreover, the district hospitals have a special public health unit, and the staff of this unit spend about 10% of their time supervising CHWs.

- In-service training is not carried out as a formal activity in the CHW programme. Instead, informal training and advice are given during supervisory visits and in regular management meetings. The cost of this type of training is not available separately.

- For various reasons the CHWs do not keep written records of their activities in the villages. Nor do they keep demographic or epidemiological records. All village-related information (data on vaccination, maternal and child health, births/deaths, and demographic and other data derived from census) is kept and updated at the health centres. The staff spend about 20 staff days per year or 5% of their time on record-keeping and data management.

- The village drug fund is a central element of the CHW programme. About half the villages have a drug fund. These funds are allowed to buy drugs at wholesale prices from the government (distribution and handling charges are not included in the price). However, because of the variety of sources (health centres, some local drug stores, district hospitals, the PCMO) and distribution patterns it is not possible to make a complete estimate of the cost of the support given to the drug funds. Only where the health services are directly involved in the distribution of the drugs is it possible to analyse the use of resources. In the PCMO pharmaceutical division, 180 days or 30% of staff time are spent on setting up drug funds and organizing logistics for one district in Lamphun Province. To transport drugs from the PCMO to the health centres, one day per month of vehicle use is needed; thereafter, each health centre needs one day per month to distribute the drugs.

- The costs for vehicle use in relation to the CHW programme, especially for supervision and drug distribution, are considerable. On an average, government drivers are used for 120 days per year and vehicles for close to 20 000 kilometres per year. In addition, 100 000 motor cycle kilometres per year at the health centre level and another 12 000 kilometres at the district level are travelled for the CHW programme.

- The cost of the CHWs' right to free medical care was also calculated. CHWs seek treatment at health centres on average 1.3 times a year and they are hospitalized once every 14 years. The average cost of health centre treatment is 15 baht, and the average cost of hospital treatment is 300 baht. Consequently, the annual cost per CHW would amount to 40.5 baht (about US$ 1.65).

To sum up, in the Lamphun Province, 5% of the PCMO staff time is spent on planning and management of the CHW programme. In addition, the work group of the PCMO pharmaceutical division devotes part of its time to organizing and supporting drug funds. At district level, the DHO staff spend 8.5% of their time on CHW-related activities (mainly supervision), and the staff of the public health unit in the district hospitals give 10% of their time to management and supervision of CHWs. At the health centre, 19% of staff time is spent on CHW-related activities, including 12% on supervision, 5% on record-keeping, 1.75% on meetings and 0.3% on drug logistics. There are also significant costs for transport.

Although a considerable amount of health personnel time and material resources are used to support the CHW programme, most of this support is not provided for in the primary health care budget established for the programme. The support activities are carried out by staff at different levels of the health system as part of their normal duties. Although, in many cases, no records are available to determine the exact amount of time spent by support staff, it proved possible to make approximate estimates of the cost of these activities on the basis of interviews with health staff and analysis of job descriptions and activity records.

Costs of the CHW programme in Jamaica[1]

Of the 1990–91 recurrent health budget of Jamaica, 18.7% was spent on primary health care services (health centres and community health aides). At national level, the costs of the community health aide programme are around 2.5% of the total health budget and 3% of the recurrent health budget. In 1990, the salaries of the aides made up 7.6% of total health personnel salaries. The government per capita expenditure on health was the equivalent of US$ 45, while the per capita expenditure of the community health aide programme in the study area was around US$ 1.24.

Of the total investment costs in the community health aide programme in the period 1972–1990, proportions of expenditure were as follows: equipment (47.8%), salaries (23.8%), travel (18.5%), and materials and supplies (10%). Of these investments, 66.2% were generated at national level and 33.8% at the regional and the parish levels. The average investment cost for the 1200 aides who were trained initially was US$ 157.

The investment costs of the programme were low because much of the initial work was done in pilot programmes developed and funded by the Department of Social and Preventive Medicine of the University of

---

[1] The information presented in this section is based on the report of a study undertaken by Dr Wolfgang Weber, University of Heidelberg, Germany, on the costs of the community health aide programme in Hanover parish, Cornwall Country Health Region, Jamaica, in 1990.

the West Indies in the late 1960s. The expenditures on these pilot programmes are not included in the investment costs calculated here. Likewise, the use of vehicles, buildings and medical equipment—other than those directly related to the training of the aides—have not been taken into account. Furthermore, the cost of teaching topics related to community health aides in basic and postgraduate training courses for nurses and midwives is not known. The inclusion of this cost would probably not change the result significantly.

The total recurrent costs of the programme in Hanover parish in the financial year 1989–90 amounted to some US\$ 108 237. This corresponds to 21.3% of the recurrent primary health care budget for the parish. The average recurrent cost per aide in the parish was US\$ 3093. These recurrent costs related to clinic work (48.2%), home visits (22.5%), general administration (13.3%), in-service training (10.2%) and supervision (5.7%). The costs appeared under the following categories in the budget: salaries (91.1%), travel (4.8%), equipment (3.8%), and material and supplies (0.3%). Recurrent costs are generated mainly at the local level (86.4%); they are insignificant at the national level (0.5%) and small at the regional or parish level (13%).

The community health aides spend about half of their total working time on clinic activities; another 30% is spent on home visits (an average of 486 hours per year), while 20% is spent on other field activities. In the Hanover parish, a community health aide makes between 9 and 39 home visits per week, or an average of 72 visits per month.

Despite the reduced scope and level of activity of the Jamaican community health aide programme in 1990 (as compared to the 1970s and the early 1980s) and the limitations of any health care programme that relies on lay personnel with minimal training, the Jamaican programme appears to be very cost-effective.

Financing mechanisms

CHW programmes are financed through various combinations of government, private sector, community and individual (fee-for-service) support. Government support has received the most attention as national programmes have started.

Government support

The government's ability to assume the costs of CHW programmes varies according to the state of the national or regional economy. In Indonesia the rural health system may be able to provide the basic resources needed but may not be able to handle the more complex management demands. The ability of the staff to continually support the CHWs was reportedly strained by the numbers of CHWs and their dispersion. In

Guinea-Bissau, government expenditure on health in 1983 was estimated to be US$2 per capita for the rural population. The recurrent costs of one CHW programme consumed most of this amount, providing only a limited range of primary health care. This neglects the need for higher-level care and population-oriented public health interventions. Thus, CHW programmes may be lower cost, but not necessarily cheap or affordable (60).

Although many governments have contributed to the investment and recurrent costs of CHW programmes in areas such as training, supervision, drugs, supplies, equipment and transport, the actual costs are commonly underestimated. Governments have assumed that a shift in emphasis from clinic-based to CHW services would result in an expansion of primary health care at low cost. As a result, governments have often not allocated enough resources for national CHW programmes.

Studies of the costs of national CHW programmes have taken place but they are difficult to carry out and to compare across countries or regions, and many of the critical expenses are the most difficult to ascertain and are based on questionable assumptions. With a lack of reliable information on how much functional areas should cost, governments continue to budget on the basis of the previous year's experience, perceptions of the current resource environment and, perhaps more importantly, current political priorities and policies in primary health care.

The influences on resource allocation to areas of health care are complex and cannot be dealt with in detail here. They include the interests of donors, political representatives, Ministry of Health leadership and special interest groups. As long as CHW programmes enjoy political priority and emphasis, it may be possible to access sufficient funds for them (see Box 11). However, even if priority is accorded to CHWs, the drive to attain an annual disease control target may supplant that priority when it comes to allocating resources.

Community support

Community participation in health development implies that communities are to be self-reliant in supporting health services, yet there is often a misunderstanding between self-reliance and self-sufficiency. Many communities will not be able to pay the total cost of CHW programmes, although many actually do support programme elements either in kind or in cash. However, given the uncertainty of many economies, such support has proved to be unreliable as a means of defraying the operational expenses of CHW programmes on a consistent basis. Moreover, in very poor communities, which may be disproportionately served by CHWs and may disproportionately utilize them too, such contributions are rarely substantial and growth potential is limited (2, 54).

63

BOX 11

Adequate resource allocation reflects political commitment

There is a notable contrast between the Chinese CHW programme and the others. This is especially striking as the Chinese programme was often cited as a model. The unique conditions of social organization in China have often been cited as essential to the success of this programme, and the lack of them has been seen as a constraint on its replication elsewhere. A further and even more striking fact is the high level of resources invested in the Chinese programme. While barefoot doctors are not civil servants, they are essentially salaried paramedics serving populations of about 500 people. This would be equivalent to having a full-time health post with qualified staff in every village in some countries. The real resources expended in training, supplies, salaries and supervision to support this system are well beyond those used elsewhere to support volunteer CHWs with several weeks of training and a minimal initial drug supply. The barefoot doctor system was established within an economy not appreciably better off than that of many other low-income nations, which suggests that political commitment, not finance, may be the main constraint in many countries.

Source: Berman et al. (*6*).

In programmes in which CHWs are salaried, lack of community contribution may be due to their being perceived as employees of the government. Communities expect government services to be delivered free. In programmes in which CHWs are volunteers, lack of community support may derive from lack of understanding of roles and responsibilities, from lack of community ownership and decision-making, or from poorly conceived and poorly implemented cost recovery schemes. In either kind of programme, CHWs may provide services that are neither expected nor valued, or their activities may simply be unreliable and lack credibility.

In order to increase funds, many communities have implemented income-generating and cost-recovery activities. The most common of these is a revolving fund for drugs. Other fund raising activities that have been tried include fees for CHW services, fees for use of a water point, poultry breeding, carpentry, tailoring and grain collection. Although some of these projects have been successful, they normally do not generate benefits that are large enough to maintain functioning CHW programmes (*54*). In Benin, attempts were made to collect funds through the sale of drugs to villagers at a modest price. The income was intended to finance the renewal of supplies, the operating cost of the village health unit and some payment to the CHWs. After several years the income was still modest and had contributed only to financing the construction of wells in villages (*11*).

Community financing schemes may also place new burdens on CHWs by requiring them to maintain accounts, to report to the community on use of funds, and even to take responsibility for misuse that they may be unable to control.

Reliance on community financing may run counter to the principle of equity in health care. It has been shown to aggravate existing inequalities within communities and between communities because of the disproportionate spread of health problems and differences in access to alternative care (54). Some villagers are more able than others to pay fees for services and for drugs, and wealthy communities will develop better health services than poor communities. Consequently, poor communities which do not receive sufficient external support may lack even the most basic care. In addition, availability of resources from communities may fluctuate considerably from year to year. In the Gambia one study uncovered considerable numbers of villagers with malaria but without the money to buy chloroquine from the village health worker. Several years of drought had diminished the availability of cash, and what little they had was being spent on food.

The development of schemes to improve the supply of drugs and generate income has been the most common approach to community financing. However, these schemes can skew the focus of primary health care systems and may introduce problems of ensuring equitable treatment. The use of profits from drug sales to pay CHWs' salaries reinforces their dispensing role rather than the primary health care approach.

As part of the health system, CHWs may supply services that people ask for or they may provide preventive services that are needed from a public health perspective but for which there is no demand. Most programmes tend to provide curative care that may be less effective in the long term but is asked for, at the expense of important preventive and promotive activities. In other cases, CHWs may be denied a curative role that would provide them with the credibility to undertake more preventive and promotive activities. Even when curative care is provided by CHWs, it may be perceived as being of lower quality and utility than that which is available from health care providers with more training.

What services do people think they need and want? Where do they want them delivered and by whom? What are the quality characteristics of these services that people expect and for which they will pay, whether in time or in money? Much has been written recently about the decreasing utilization of CHWs. Why utilization is decreasing may relate to the disjunction between health beliefs and felt needs, changing epidemiological patterns, and the intended role and training of the CHWs (8). It may also be related to inadequacies in the systems that support and supply CHWs with what they need to provide quality services (6).

Matching community ideas of CHW services with what is both feasible and useful from the perspective of the health system might facilitate decision-making about where to allocate resources. How can CHW programmes improve understanding of and develop appropriate demand for services? How can programmes use this information to encourage adequate allocation of resources?

Other private sector support

Community financing is at best only a part of the development of the economic viability of CHW programmes. Other factors include the support of NGOs and international organizations as well as of multilateral and bilateral donors. Donor agencies primarily support specific time-limited projects and their contributions do not sustain national health programmes. Nonetheless, sometimes donor influence and interests may skew government or community priorities. The role of the private sector in financing such programmes is less well understood. NGOs have been able to establish and sustain CHW programmes, generally in clearly-defined geographic areas. It is reasonable to assume that governments working in partnership with NGOs can negotiate shared financing of CHWs. However, there are risks, as illustrated in the evolution of the Zimbabwean village health worker programme, where increasing professionalization of village health workers and conflicts in authority and accountability between the government, the NGO and communities essentially undermined early successes.

The potential roles of private sector health care providers, such as traditional healers and private practitioners, and of pharmacies or industries, in financing or supporting CHW programmes have yet to be extensively explored. While private providers or enterprises are unlikely to play a national role, they are increasingly important at local level. As countries become more industrialized and urbanized, the role of the private sector may grow and the potential role of CHWs in it should be studied. For the time being, it is reasonable to expect that governments that want CHW programmes will have to pay for them.

Resource allocation

Government decision-making on the allocation of resources in the health sector has influenced the effectiveness of CHW programmes and constrained their potential for improving health. As governments have become increasingly interested in the cost–effectiveness of interventions, focused disease control programmes have taken priority. Typically, CHW programmes have been seen as distinct interventions like EPI and CDD. In this context, the costs of CHWs may have seemed high compared to the costs of disease control because the budgeting process of disease control programmes fails to take account of the demands of the programmes on the mainstays of the health services delivery system—personnel time and logistic support. National EPI and CDD programmes have specific, measurable targets and the cost of elements such as vaccine, ORS, training and the collection of information must have seemed clear and distinct.

However, CHWs are not separate. They are part of the service capacity. Yet in the minds of budget decision-makers, they are competing for scarce resources to develop capacity. EPI, CDD and other focused disease interventions have made extensive use of CHWs to achieve their own objectives—without any contribution to the cost of the CHWs' time and effort. The cost–effectiveness figures for EPI underestimate the resource burden placed on CHWs and communities alike. The costs of CHWs, which may contribute horizontally to the achievement of all disease control objectives, are not equated with the effects attributed to disease control.

Resource support to CHWs is an investment in the capacity of the health system. CHWs can participate in many formerly vertical activities and improve their effectiveness. As decentralization and community involvement in health increases, it will become clear that CHWs are not an alternative programme but an integral part of a long-term strategy to improve public health. The documented effectiveness of CHWs in the areas of prevention and promotion, and their utility across levels of economic development, should make it clear that they are not simply a solution for the poor. CHW programmes have progressed a long way from the time when they were considered stop-gap measures and have since demonstrated their potential to improve health.

In making decisions about what resources to invest in health service delivery, it is important to assess and compare the supply of health services and community demands and expectations in the context of public health goals. CHWs are a means for capacity-building and service provision within that environment and governments can decide to invest in them. What is essential is that CHWs must have adequate resources, just like any other programme, in order to reach their full potential.

CHAPTER 4

Conclusion: the way forward

The world is being challenged to respond to new health problems, emerging diseases, and economic, political and cultural changes. As technology becomes more complex, and as health systems do not seem to result in improved health, there is much talk of the need for "health reform". What is the way forward for CHW programmes in this rapidly changing environment?

The issues and questions relating to CHWs are currently being discussed in the wider context of the debate on health reform. Changes in people's health and in the patterns of disease, political changes with increasing emphasis on decentralization, the ever-growing cost of health care and the ever-diminishing prospect of universal access to it, and the demands of free market economies are all critical elements in this debate. Against this background, strategies for health sector reform will vary from country to country. However, a number of common elements in this move towards reform are beginning to emerge. First, the role of government is expected to change from that of the provider of health services to that of regulator of such services in an open and competitive market. Health is likely to be seen in economic terms, as a commodity whose supply and quality will depend upon the financial resources of the purchaser. Second, the decentralization of government health services is seen as potentially the most critical need in order both to improve efficiency and also to ensure that the services respond to local health needs and conditions. Third, new ways of financing health care and services will be crucial if current health services are not to be crushed by increasing costs and the imperative need to make basic services available to all.

The push for major reforms on the lines of the above is relatively recent, but already the protagonists are taking sides. In particular, there are concerns about placing on the shoulder of the poor the burden for the costs of health care, about the consequences of increasing privatization of medical services, and about the implication that reduced government spending could result in a move from a comprehensive to a narrower and more selective approach to health care. There are few models and strategies appropriate to developed countries that are inappropriate in less developed ones. While the overburdening costs of health care provision may be the critical issue in one country, in another

68

the issue may have more to do with availability of care. If health care and development are given up to market forces—and good use and efficiency of economic resources are key issues in this move—it is unclear what the future roles of human resources will be.

Perhaps the most serious danger in the current international push for health sector reform is that governments, and particularly those of least developed countries, are placing too much hope on the promise of new resource schemes (privatization, community financing, increasing or introducing user charges, insurance, etc.), while in reality it may not be possible to implement these schemes meaningfully in those largely subsistence economies. Some governments are busy introducing and managing these schemes at the expense of perennially urgent needs such as rationalizing existing health expenditure and shifting extra resources to health from such areas as defence and security.

In the context of well-supported CHW programmes therefore, proposals for health sector reform need to be considered against the background of the overwhelming inability of resource-poor countries and desperately poor people either to provide meaningful services or to pay for their primary health care needs.

Organizational reforms such as decentralization hold greater potential for CHW programmes. It has been argued in this book that the most promising organizational reform would be the creation or strengthening of district health systems based on primary health care principles. The big question is what will happen to CHW programmes where health services are expected or encouraged to operate in open and competitive markets. Would CHWs continue to be community workers supported by public funds and structures or would they be private workers with private funds and structures?

There is no question that CHWs are essential. What should be clear from this review is that the problems of CHW programmes are the same as the problems of health services. These problems have been extensively studied and discussed, and reasonable solutions are proposed. The challenges that face the proponents of these programmes now are not when and why and how to go about making them work—but actually moving forward with the hard work of implementation.

References

1. The World Bank. *World development report, 1993. Investing in health.* New York, Oxford University Press, 1993.

2. *Strengthening the performance of community health workers in primary health care. Report of a WHO Study Group.* Geneva, World Health Organization, 1989 (WHO Technical Report Series, No. 780).

3. *Lessons without borders. Immunization: making it work at home and abroad.* Washington, DC, United States Agency for International Development, 1994.

4. *Better health in Africa. Experiences and lessons learned.* Washington, DC, World Bank, 1994.

5. Walt G. *Community health workers in national programmes. Just another pair of hands?* Milton Keynes, Open University Press, 1990.

6. Berman PA, Gwatkin DR, Burger SE. Community based health workers: head start or false start towards health for all? *Social science and medicine,* 1987, 25(5):443–459.

7. Frankel S, ed. *The community health worker. Effective programmes for developing countries.* Oxford, Oxford University Press, 1992.

8. de Geyndt W, Zhoa X, Liu S. *From barefoot doctor to village doctor in rural China.* Washington, DC, World Bank, 1992 (World Bank Technical Paper, No. 187).

9. Zhu N et al. Factors associated with the decline of the Cooperative Medical System and barefoot doctors in rural China. *Bulletin of the World Health Organization,* 1989, 67(4):431–441.

10. *Local government focused acceleration of primary health care. The Nigerian experience. Report of a WHO review.* Geneva, World Health Organization, 1992 (unpublished document SHS/DHS/92.1; available on request from Division of Analysis, Research and Assessment, World Health Organization, 1211 Geneva 27, Switzerland).

11. *Strengthening the performance of community health workers: Interregional Meeting of Principal Investigators, 12–16 November 1990, Geneva, Switzerland.* Geneva, World Health Organization, 1990 (unpublished document SHS/DHS/91.1; available on request from Division of Analysis, Research and Assessment, World Health Organization, 1211 Geneva 27, Switzerland).

12. *The challenge of implementation. District health systems for primary health care.* Geneva, World Health Organization, 1988 (unpublished document SHS/DHS/88.1; available on request from Division of Analysis, Research and Assessment, World Health Organization, 1211 Geneva 27, Switzerland).

13. Sanders D. The state of democratization in primary health care: community participation and the village health worker programme in Zimbabwe. In: Frankel S, ed. *The community health worker. Effective programmes for developing countries*. Oxford, Oxford University Press, 1992:178–219.

14. Gray HH, Ciroma J. Reducing attribution among village health workers in rural Nigeria. *Socio-economic planning and science*, 1988, 22(1):39–43.

15. Walt G et al. Are large-scale volunteer community health worker programmes feasible? The case of Sri Lanka. *Social science and medicine*, 1989, 29(5):599–608.

16. *Health manpower requirements for the achievement of health for all by the year 2000 through primary health care. Report of a WHO Study Group*. Geneva, World Health Organization, 1985 (WHO Technical Report Series, No. 717).

17. Otti PN. Medical education and primary health care in tropical Africa: evidence for change. *East African medical journal*, 1989, 66(4):300–306.

18. Chabot HT, Bremmers J. Government health services versus community: conflict or harmony? *Social science and medicine*, 1988, 26(9):957–962.

19. Ebrahim GJ et al. Learning from doing: progression to primary health care within a national health programme. A case study from Tanzania. *Journal of tropical paediatrics*, 1988, 34(1):4–11, 1988.

20. Walt G. Community health workers: are national programmes in crisis? *Health policy and planning*, 1988, 3(1):1–21.

21. Burbano E et al. *Community health workers in Colombia: is preventive care sufficient?* London, London School of Hygiene and Tropical Medicine, 1988.

22. Knudsen T et al. *Family welfare educators in Botswana: can they be more community oriented?* London, London School of Hygiene and Tropical Medicine, 1988.

23. Katz FM, Fülöp T, eds. *Personnel for health care: case studies of educational programmes*. Geneva, World Health Organization, 1978 (Public Health Papers, No. 70).

24. Braveman PA, Mora F. Training physicians for community-oriented primary care in Latin America: model programmes in Mexico, Nicaragua and Costa Rica. *American journal of public health*, 1987, 77(4):485–490.

25. Waterston T, Sanders D. Teaching primary health care: some lessons from Zimbabwe. *Medical education*, 1987, 21:4–9.

26. Joseph A. Training doctors for primary health care: the Vellore model. *World health forum*, 1985, 6:118–121.

27. Paine LHW, Siem Tjam F. *Hospitals and the health care revolution*. Geneva, World Health Organization, 1988.

28. DeBoer CN, McNeil M. Hospital outreach community-based health care: the case of Chogoria, Kenya. *Social science and medicine*, 1989, 28(10):1007–1017.

29. Jacobson ML et al. A case study of the Tenwek hospital community health programme in Kenya. *Social science and medicine*, 1989, 28(10):1059–1062.

30. Matomora MK. A people-centred approach to primary health care implementation in Mvumi, Tanzania. *Social science and medicine*, 1989, 28(10):1031–1037.

31. *Community health workers: pillars for health for all. Report of the Interregional Conference, Yaoundé, Cameroon, 1–5 December 1986.* Geneva, World Health Organization 1987 (unpublished document SHS/CIH/87.2; available on request from Division of Analysis, Research and Assessment, World Health Organization, 1211 Geneva 27, Switzerland).

32. *The role of civil society in district health systems: hidden resources.* Geneva, World Health Organization, 1996 (unpublished document WHO/ARA/96.3; available on request from Division of Analysis, Research and Assessment, World Health Organization, 1211 Geneva 27, Switzerland).

33. *Education for health. A manual on health education in primary health care.* Geneva, World Health Organization, 1988.

34. Bentley C. Primary health care in northwestern Somalia. A case study. *Social science and medicine*, 1989, 28(10):1019–1030.

35. Mangelsdorf KR. The selection and training of primary health care workers in Ecuador: issues and alternatives for public policy. *International journal of health services*, 1988, 18(3):471–493.

36. Mburu FM. Whither community-based health care? *Social science and medicine*, 1989, 28(10):1073–1079.

37. Kaseje D, Sempebwa E. An integrated rural health project in Saradidi, Kenya. *Social science and medicine*, 1989, 28(10):1063–1071.

38. Tumwine JK. Community participation as myth or reality: a personal experience from Zimbabwe. *Health policy and planning*, 1989, 4(2):157–161.

39. Madan TN. Community involvement in health policy: socio-structural and dynamic aspects of health beliefs. *Social science and medicine*, 1987, 25(6):615–620.

40. Cham K et al. Social organization and political factionalism: PHC in the Gambia. *Health policy and planning*, 1987, 2(3):214–226.

41. Cooray NT. Decentralization of health services in Sri Lanka. In: Mills A et al, eds. *Health system decentralization.* Geneva, World Health Organization, 1990.

42. Kaseje D. Community-based health care: the Saradidi, Kenya, experience. In: Halstead SB, Walsh JA, eds. *Why things work. Case histories in development. Proceedings of a conference held in Bellagio, Italy, October 26–31, 1987.* Boston, Adams Publishing Group, 1990.

43. Laleman G, Annys S. Understanding community participation: a health programme in the Philippines. *Health policy and planning*, 1989, 4(3):251–256.

44. UNICEF. *The state of the world's children, 1987.* New York, Oxford University Press, 1987.

45. McConnel C, Taylor M. Community health workers in Nepal. In: Frankel S, ed. *The community health worker. Effective programmes for developing countries.* Oxford, Oxford University Press, 1992:102–124.

46. UNICEF. *The state of the world's children, 1988.* New York, Oxford University Press, 1988.

47. Ofosu-Aamah V. *National experience in the use of community health workers. A review of current issues and problems.* Geneva, World Health Organization, 1983 (WHO Offset Publication, No. 71).

48. Hope R, Carter CA, Rai IM. Utilizing education infrastructure for primary health care. *Tropical doctor*, 1988, 18(1):37–39.

49. Lengeler C et al. Rapid, low-cost two-step method to screen for urinary schistosomiasis at the district level: the Kilosa experience. *Bulletin of the World Health Organization*, 1991, 69:179–189.

50. Ghai D. *Participatory development: some perspectives from grassroots experiences.* Geneva, United Nations Research Institute for Social Development, 1988 (Discussion paper, No. 5).

51. Kaseje DC, Sempebwa EK, Spencer HC. Community leadership and participation in the Saradidi, Kenya, rural health development programme. *Annals of tropical medicine and parasitology*, 1987, 81(Suppl.1):46–55.

52. Walt G et al. Community health workers in national programmes: the case of the family welfare educators of Botswana. *Transactions of the Royal Society of Tropical Medicine and Hygiene*, 1989, 83(1):49–55.

53. Stone L. Primary health care for whom? Village perspectives from Nepal. *Social science and medicine*, 1986, 22(3):293–302.

54. Abel-Smith B, Dua A. Community financing in developing countries: the potential for the health sector. *Health policy and planning*, 1988, 3(2):95–108.

55. Hongvivatana T et al. *Alternatives to primary health care volunteers in Thailand.* Bangkok, Mahidol University, 1988 (Monograph Series, No. 5).

56. *Traditional healers as community health workers.* Geneva, World Health Organization, 1991 (unpublished document WHO/SHS/DHS/91.6; available on request from Division of Analysis, Research and Assessment, World Health Organization, 1211 Geneva 27, Switzerland).

57. Health for all: from words to deeds. *World health forum*, 1987, 8(2):164–183.

58. *Community involvement in health development: challenging health services. Report of a WHO Study Group.* Geneva, World Health Organization, 1991 (WHO Technical Report Series, No. 809)

59. Briceno-Leon R. Rural housing for control of Chagas disease in Venezuela. *Parasitology today*, 1987, 3(12):384–387.

60. Chabot J, Waddington C. Primary health care is not cheap: a case study from Guinea Bissau. *International journal of health services*, 1987, 17(3):387–409.